SUPER IMMUNITY

SUPER IMMUNITY

The Essential Nutrition Guide
for Boosting Your Body's Defenses to Live
Longer, Stronger, and Disease Free

Joel Fuhrman, M.D.

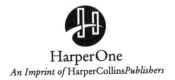

HarperOne
An Imprint of HarperCollins*Publishers*

HarperOne

SUPER IMMUNITY: *The Essential Nutrition Guide for Boosting Your Body's Defenses to Live Longer, Stronger, and Disease Free.* Copyright © 2011 by Joel Fuhrman, M.D. All rights reserved. Printed in the United States of America. No part of this book may be used or reproduced in any manner whatsoever without written permission except in the case of brief quotations embodied in critical articles and reviews. For information address HarperCollins Publishers, 10 East 53rd Street, New York, NY 10022.

HarperCollins books may be purchased for educational, business, or sales promotional use. For information please write: Special Markets Department, HarperCollins Publishers, 10 East 53rd Street, New York, NY 10022.

HarperCollins website: http://www.harpercollins.com

HarperCollins®, 📖®, and HarperOne™ are trademarks of HarperCollins Publishers

FIRST HARPERCOLLINS PAPERBACK EDITION PUBLISHED IN 2012

Interior Design by Laura Lind Design
Photos used with permission of the author.
Illustrations by Savita Naidu.

Library of Congress Cataloging-in-Publication Data is available upon request.

ISBN 978–0–06–208064–6

13 14 15 16 17 RRD(H) 10 9 8 7 6 5 4 3 2 1

Dedicated to my wife, Lisa, whose encouragement and love have enabled me to pursue my dreams.

Contents

INTRODUCTION: What Is Super Immunity?   1

ONE   Food Equals Health   11

TWO   The Failure of Modern Medicine   37

THREE   Super Foods for Super Immunity   57

FOUR   Cold and Flu—What We Need to Know   85

FIVE   Healthy Carbs, Fats, and Proteins   109

SIX   Making the Right Choices   135

SEVEN   Menus and Recipes   175

GLOSSARY   247

NOTES   255

ACKNOWLEDGMENTS   279

INDEX   281

What Is Super Immunity?

*It just dawned on me that two and a half years ago I began
the wonderful journey with you to get my health back, and I
did not just lose one hundred pounds; I haven't had a virus,
cold, or flu bug since. Considering that for over thirty years
straight I would get a nasty case of bronchitis every winter
and I'd cough like crazy for six weeks, this freedom truly is
wonderful—in more ways than just preventing obesity, cancer, type 2 diabetes, and heart disease.*

—Emily Boller

Super Immunity can be best defined as the body's immune system
working to its fullest potential. Modern science has advanced to the
point where we have evidence that the right raw materials and nutritional factors can double or triple the protective power of the immune
system. If you learn to fill every cell receptor lock with the right nutrient key and meet the demands of each cell, the body's defenses take
on superhero qualities—and you will hardly ever get sick again. More
important, this change from average immunity to Super Immunity can
save your life.

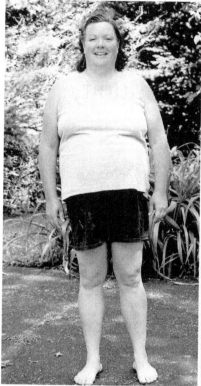
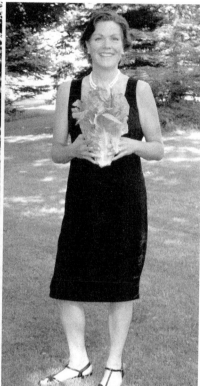

Emily Boller, July 2008.   *June 2009.*

The fact is that Super Immunity is needed now, more than ever. In the United States, adults can expect to catch a cold two to four times a year, and children can expect to get six to ten colds annually. All of these colds sap about $40 billion from the U.S. economy in direct and indirect costs. On top of that, getting sick is no fun. Influenza, for example, can result in a prolonged and serious illness. With health authorities' warnings about the potential of new flu epidemics and the global spread of viral illnesses, it is vital that we keep our immune system strong and know the steps to take to protect ourselves and our families. In someone without a well-functioning immune system, a mild infection can hang on for weeks; worse yet, it can develop serious consequences such as heart damage or nerve paralysis, or it can blossom into a difficult-to-treat bacterial infection such as a life-threatening pneumonia.

Our immune system also protects us from developing cancer. The same white blood cells and other immune system components that are utilized to fight infection are also used to recognize our own human cells as they become abnormal and to remove them before they can evolve into a tumor or cancer.

The immune system is like an angel watching over our lives and protecting us from the risks around us. With Super Immunity you can have a healthier, happier life with more comfort and productivity. Super Immunity can also enable you to push the envelope of human longevity, because it puts a force field of protection around the body, radically reducing the risk of annoying minor infections, serious major infections, and even cancers.

Today we are exposed to more dangerous infections from around the world than ever before. We are routinely in airports and jets crowded with world travelers who have come in contact with exotic and newly created microbes, and we are in schools and hospitals with bacteria circulating that have developed antibiotic resistance. Scientists suggest that environmental, social, and nutritional changes have helped trigger an unprecedented explosion of infection: more than thirty-five new infectious diseases have burst upon the world in the past thirty years. The U.S. death rate from infectious diseases is now double what it was in 1980, up to 170,000 annually. With two billion people traveling by air each year, the potential for serious viral illnesses looms even larger in our future.[1]

Once a disease takes hold these days, it tends to be globalized quickly by travel and trade. The West Nile virus, for example, is thought to have reached New York from its traditional home in the Middle East on an infected bird carried by a ship or a plane. Within six weeks after SARS (severe acute respiratory syndrome) first appeared in November 2002, it had spread worldwide, carried by unsuspecting travelers. According to the World Health Organization (WHO), 8,000 people were infected with this severe viral illness, and about 800 eventually died during the outbreak.[2] This will certainly not be the last viral illness to travel from one region of the globe to another, spreading rapidly to highly populated areas, but it set a record for speed of continent-to-continent transmission.

In addition to the increased risk of dangerous infections circling the globe, we have another modern epidemic affecting a large segment of our population: cancer. The lifetime probability of being diagnosed with an invasive cancer is 44 percent for men and 37 percent for women. However, because of the earlier median age of diagnosis for breast cancer compared with other major cancers, women have a slightly higher probability of developing cancer before the age of sixty. Currently, one in four deaths in the United States is due to cancer. The statistical trend for women looks bleak: breast cancer, almost unheard of a hundred years ago, now affects one in eight women over their lifetime, with signs that this may increase in the next few decades.

Together, we can turn these statistical trends around. Research from the field of nutritional medicine has shown us that there is a clear way to improve and sustain our health and fight off illness in all its forms.

I believe that the nutritional research and information in these pages is essential and needs to become common knowledge. The modern diet is causing a tragic reduction in immune competency. Due to the increase in consumption of processed foods, "fake" foods, food additives, and all the cancer-causing elements these things contain, our current food environment is compromising our health. We must intercede with relevant research from nutritional science and empower people to protect themselves *before* we see the continued degradation of our daily health; *before* a massive life-threatening epidemic explodes; and *before* we witness a secondary explosive wave of cancer.

Super Immunity is well within our reach. Before we talk about *how*, it is important for you to learn about immune system competency and what it can do for you and your health.

More Medical Care, *Not* the Answer

We are living in an era of rapid advancements in science, and much of this new knowledge can be applied to help us live better, longer, and happier than ever before. But let me warn you: exposure to more medical care, more drugs, more vaccines, and more doctors does *not* beget Super Immunity. In fact, medical care is part of the problem, not the solution.

When most of us think of preventive medicine and proper health care, we think about getting shots, taking medications, or having diagnostic tests. We've had these products and services marketed to us for the last fifty years and have accepted a belief system that equates more medical care with better health, survival, and longevity. This equation is simply not true.

As a matter of fact, the Kaiser Health Foundation, which studied this issue in depth, determined that one-third of medical spending is devoted to services that don't improve health or the quality of care—and may make things worse![3] Too many people are becoming sicker and sicker. A *lack* of medical care is not the problem, and *more* medical care is certainly not the answer.

The new patients I see daily in my practice are great examples. People may catch a cold or flu that lingers for weeks, and then have a cough that lingers for additional months. Often we see patients develop facial headaches from a sinusitis that lasts for months after a simple cold. The most minor illnesses turn into major calamities requiring more and more medications. The medications may help initially, but after a while they stop working and the initial problem reappears, often worse than before. These medical complications occur because of impaired natural immunity that results from a combination of inadequate nutrition and medications that have degraded our body's ability to protect itself.

Laura Kaminski is a wonderful example of how proper nutrition can repair the immune system, making it stronger than ever before. Laura, a former patient of mine, wrote to me about her experience:

> *I was allergic to pollen, grass, trees, ragweed, and cats, and was chronically congested. After being on antihistamines, and needing antibiotics over and over again, I developed recurrent UTIs [urinary tract infections] and bacterial sinus infections. I tried one diet after another to try to lose weight too; I craved food and felt guilty about my eating habits. It was a roller-coaster ride of one illness after another and more and more drugs—and I was still in my thirties.*
>
> *Finally, after I read your work, it began to all make sense; I realized my immune system was weak. I dropped the fifteen pounds I had been trying to lose for years, and within weeks I felt mentally sharper and my stomach stopped bothering me. The really exciting part came six months later, when I realized my allergies were gone. I could finally breathe freely again and my allergies, sinus infections, and frequent urinary tract infections simply disappeared. I no longer need drugs anymore. I have discovered what really works to stay in great health, and that settles it for me.*

What Laura experienced is available to all of us. This new science that you are going to learn in the subsequent pages is too valuable to remain hidden in the basement library of a medical school. Everybody needs to know that they can transform their lives too.

What most of us are still unaware of is how a weakened immunity, common to those eating the standard American diet, leaves us more exposed.

Not only does a weakened immune system leave us vulnerable to influenza and other diseases, but we have evidence to indicate that our overuse of antibiotics and other medications may be a contributory factor in the development of cancer.

A study published in the *Journal of the American Medical Association* (*JAMA*) provides evidence that the use of antibiotics is associated with an increased risk of breast cancer. Authors from the National Cancer Institute (a part of the National Institutes of Health in Bethesda, Maryland), the University of Washington in Seattle, and the Fred Hutchinson Cancer Center, also in Seattle, concluded that the more antibiotics the women in the study used, the higher their risk of breast cancer.[4]

The authors of this *JAMA* study found that women who'd had more than twenty-five prescriptions—over an average period of seventeen years—had more than twice the risk of breast cancer than women who had not taken any antibiotics. However, even women who had between one and twenty-five prescriptions over that same period had an increased risk; they were about one and a half times more likely to be diagnosed with breast cancer than women who hadn't taken any antibiotics. The authors found an increased risk in all classes of antibiotics that they studied.

I remember the first pharmacology lecture I heard in medical school, when the professor emphasized, "Make no doubt about it: all drugs are toxic and can even hasten one's death. They should be used only after careful consideration of the risk-to-benefit ratio, because they all have considerable and serious risks." Couple our nutrient-poor diet—and the resultant immune system weaknesses, leading to frequent illnesses—with the use and overuse of medications, including antibiotics, vaccines, and immunosuppressive drugs for autoimmune diseases, and we have a good reason for the explosion in cancer rates over the last seventy years. But we can alter this course.

That witches' cauldron of nutritional deficiencies coupled with the overuse and dependency on medication is destructive to our health as we age. If you, like Laura, are sick all the time, if you are overly dependent on drugs just to feel "normal," that should trigger an alarm. Those frequent infections are like your body's immunity alarm. Excellent health is not merely how you feel at the moment; it is how resistant your immune system is to microbes, which also reflects how resistant you are to cancer. This is a serious subject that may be uncomfortable to discuss, but it is too important to hide from. Laura's frequent infections and dependency on drugs finally triggered an alarm and alerted Laura. Deep down she knew she had to change. Today, with her improved health, she has protected herself in more ways than she even knows at this point. She was heading toward a health tragedy that she averted.

Protecting Yourself with Super Immunity

We were taught that viruses are passed from person to person via hand-to-face behavior but are otherwise unavoidable. If this is true, why do some of us get sick more often than others? What makes some people more susceptible? Once someone in our household or workplace is sick, are we simply doomed to get sick as well?

What if science advanced to the point where it became possible to become almost totally resistant to colds, influenza, and other infections—and if you did "catch" something, you bounced back to wellness within twenty-four hours? What if we could prevent the complications of viral and bacterial exposures and keep them as minor annoyances that never evolved into more dangerous infections? What if it were possible to develop Super Immunity to infections? Wouldn't you want to have it?

What if we found out how to build immune defenses with proper nutrition to develop Super Immunity—defenses so strong that more than 80 percent of cancers would not occur? What if these same positive actions enabled you to age more slowly and maintain your youthful vigor and excellent health into your later years?

The truth is that nutritional science has made phenomenal strides and discoveries in recent years, and if you apply this new science to your dietary choices, it will enable you to take control of your health destiny. At this point in the history of nutritional science, evidence exists demonstrating that the human immune system can be supercharged to protect our bodies against disease. I will help you understand this new science and put it into action in your kitchen and your life.

Food gives us energy and the building blocks to grow in the form of calories, but we have not fully appreciated the *noncaloric* micronutrients in food, including those that are neither vitamins nor minerals, but phytochemicals—elements that strengthen and support normal immune function. This book teaches you about these critical factors for normalizing and strengthening immune function. Utilizing a combination of foods that are rich in powerful, immunity-strengthening phytochemicals and other micronutrients, it's possible to prevent most common modern diseases. By maximizing the function and protective potential of the human immune system, we can earn Super Immunity.

Super Immunity helps with everything from the colds and flu to cancer. This is not only about getting through the flu season; it is about living with superior health *for the rest of your life*. We are not talking about just a quick fix, but an entire shift in how we understand our health and wellness.

Life is not without risks, and of course optimal nutrition cannot prevent all microbial diseases and all cancers. Nevertheless, with advancements in modern medicine, nutritional science, and microbiology, there is no reason why the most common serious diseases should not become exceedingly *un*common.

I hope you scrutinize and critique carefully the information presented in this book. I hope many of you review the scientific references listed as well, and confirm their accuracy. If you do so, I think you will find that the evidence is too great to be ignored, and the solution too delicious. Super Immunity is available for those who choose it!

CHAPTER ONE

Food Equals Health

Before I began to incorporate Dr. Fuhrman's ideas into my own diet, I was always getting colds and suffering from almost chronic sinus infections. Heck, I almost died of pneumonia twice. But now I am never sick. I haven't had a cold in three years. I track my nutritional intake and I can see for myself that I am now eating a diet that meets and exceeds the recommended intake of almost all vitamins and minerals. And now I understand why I was so sickly before: I was getting so little nutrition. Thank you, Dr. Fuhrman.

—Aram Barsamian

Historians and archaeologists have revealed that ancient civilizations all over the world recognized that certain foods could provide health-promoting and disease-protective benefits. The historically documented use of certain foods and food extracts from dried plants for healing indicates that the early application of the knowledge about the health-giving functions of plant-derived compounds dates back thousands of years.

Natural plants are complex packages of biologically active compounds. The term "phytochemicals," which means "plant-chemicals," was coined to represent these thousands of plant-sourced compounds that have functional effects in animal tissues with subtle but profound effects on human health and immunity. With the recent discovery that superior immune function in humans is dependent on a broad array of these plant-derived chemicals, we can appreciate that food supplies us not only with the basic nutritive functions, but also with a secondary level of nutrition that adds a complex layer of disease resistance and longevity benefits. These secondary benefits have not been adequately appreciated until recently.

Our evolution in a world of edible plants allowed the human body to take advantage of the complex biochemical compounds found in plants that we could use to support superior functioning of our cells. In recent years we have discovered fascinating and enormously complex interactions within our cells—interactions by which a combination of phytochemicals support defensive and self-reparative machinery we never knew the human body possessed.

Phytochemicals are bioactive, plant-derived chemical compounds important for the growth and survival of the plant; they came about for the benefit of the plant world. However, the human immune system evolved dependent on these phytochemicals for its optimal functioning. Some people, objecting to the connotations of the word "chemical" (with its connection to artificial and toxic compounds), prefer to use the word "phytonutrients," so you will often see those words interchanged. However, the word "chemical" is really what we might call agnostic, disconnected from particular dogma; and the widely established word "phytochemical" is the correct term to represent the broad array of these newly discovered compounds with complicated health effects.

Superior nutrition is the secret to Super Immunity, and it is relatively simple. It does not take years of study and contemplation to become an expert in human nutrition as long as you understand the principles that govern your basic food choices and food preparation. Just like the complicated and synergistic nature of the human immune system, natural plants are complicated and wondrous life forms; they contain thousands of intricate cells and biochemicals working in harmony. Animals and plants developed a fragile, interconnected, and symbiotic relationship on earth, and now human beings rely on plants for our health and survival. When studying the survival potential of animals and humans, we must realize that we are dependent on the health and quality of the food grown from the earth to sustain us: the health of the food we eat ultimately determines our own health. When we eat healthy food, we become healthy; when we don't, we develop disease. Essentially, we are made from the food we eat. As it is commonly said, we are what we eat.

Unfortunately, when we cultivate nutritional deficiencies in our body over long periods of time, especially in our formative years, it can create cellular damage resulting in serious illnesses in later life that can be difficult to resolve. In addition, these deficiencies result in inferior immunity.

The great news for all of us is that the recent advancements in nutritional science have created an opportunity to earn great health via what we eat. And, as you will discover, it is not only the powerful compounds in foods such as berries and pomegranates that are so protective, but these compounds—when combined with those found in green vegetables, mushrooms, and onions in the diet—fuel the miraculous self-healing and self-protective properties *already built into the human genome,* together resulting in Super Immunity.

A *combination* of these compounds is more effective than a single agent, even in a high dose. For example, taking a large dose of vitamin C or vitamin E is not very effective, especially if no deficiency existed prior to dosing. Likewise, although certain phytochemical compounds have more profound, long-acting, and powerful free-radical-scavenging effects than do known antioxidant vitamins such as C and E (more on antioxidants and free radicals later), supplementing with a hefty dose of a natural phytochemical extracted from a green vegetable would not offer as much protection as combining it with the *hundreds* of other

beneficial compounds found in nutrient-rich foods. Acting coopera-
tively, these newly identified micronutrients work together to fuel an
assortment of mechanisms that both prevent cell damage and also kill
heavily damaged cells that cannot be adequately repaired, before they
become dangerous to the body.

My "nutritarian" approach, which includes and mixes the most
powerful and protective foods in the diet, is natural, comes without
toxicity, and can prevent many human tragedies—not just revving up
our immune system against infection and cancer, but also preventing
heart attacks, strokes, and dementia.

The American Dietary Disaster, or Death from Processed Foods

Because the modern diet in America and much of the world today is
so rich in processed foods and animal products and so low in natural vegetation, especially vegetables, almost all Americans are dramatically deficient in plant-derived phytochemicals, and the effects are
far-reaching and dangerous.

Twenty-five years ago, we worshipped vitamins and minerals, and
nutritional scientists hardly knew phytochemicals existed; now those
compounds are considered the major micronutrient load in natural
foods, and their effects are recognized as broad and profound. In other
words, we now know that vitamins and minerals are not nearly enough.
To have normal immune function we require hundreds of additional
phytochemicals, found in natural plants. Supplements are appearing
in the marketplace that contain these beneficial compounds and they
show promise, but nothing can match the immunity-building power
of a diet that contains an adequate amount and broad array of these
health-enhancing substances from unrefined plant foods.

Today, the American diet takes over 60 percent of its calories from processed foods—a percentage that has increased gradually but inexorably

USA FOOD CONSUMPTION DATA

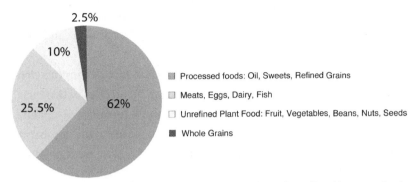

USDA Economics Research Service, 2005; www.ers.usda.gov/Data/FoodConsumption/
FoodGuideIndex.htm#calories.

over the last hundred years. This category encompasses most foods made with added sweeteners, with white flour, and with oils. Processed foods include the following: white bread, bagels, chips, pasta, donuts, cookies, breakfast bars, cold cereals, soft drinks, pretzels, condiments, and premade salad dressings. These processed foods are generally mixed with additives, coloring agents, and preservatives to extend shelf life, and they're placed in plastic bags and cardboard boxes.

Soft drinks, sugar, corn syrup, and other sweeteners now occupy a major share of the dietary pie. The amount of cheese and chicken has also increased significantly in the American diet over the last century, with the consumption of calories from animal products now at over 25 percent. With so many animal products and processed foods in the modern diet, there is little room for unrefined or unprocessed vegetation.

Americans consume less than 10 percent of their calories from unrefined plant foods such as fruits, beans, seeds, and vegetables. However, that 10 percent figure is misleading, because about half the vegetable consumption in America is white potato products, including fries and chips! If you remove the white potato from consideration (not a particularly nutritious food), the other produce would amount to less than 5 percent of the American diet.

The modern diet is not slightly deficient in just a handful of micro-nutrients; it is grossly deficient in hundreds of important plant-derived, immunity-building compounds. These are not optional; you can't have a lifetime of good health without them.

To identify these important antioxidants and phytochemicals deficient in the American diet, we must recognize a broad class of beneficial compounds, including the whole carotene family (including lycopene, beta-carotene, alpha-carotene, lutein, and zeaxanthin); and an assortment of other compounds that maximize cell function, thus enabling the healing properties of immune cells—compounds such as alpha-lipoic acid, flavonoids, bioflavonoids, polyphenols and phenolic acids, quercetin, rutin, anthocyanins and proanthocyanins, allium compounds, allyl sulfides, glucosinolates, isothiocyanates, lignans, and pectins. All these classes of compounds impact our health; and without them our health, and especially our immune system, dramatically suffers.

No matter how many different dietary theories there are out there, pretty much everyone agrees that vegetables are "good for you." But just how good they truly are has been debated. Sadly, the data from observational studies is often flawed simply because most people don't eat enough vegetables to have a measurable impact on their health! However, some long-term observational studies do indeed demonstrate that vegetable consumption is the most important factor in preventing chronic disease and premature death.[1]

The Nature and Function of Antioxidants

Since neither processed foods nor animal products contain a significant load of antioxidant nutrients or any phytochemicals, the modern diet is dramatically disease-promoting. In other words, we are eating ourselves to sickness. Antioxidants are vitamins, minerals, and phytochemicals that aid the body in removing "free radicals" and controlling free-radical production.

Why is this so important? Free radicals are molecules that contain an unpaired electron, which causes them to be highly chemically reactive. This unstable molecule is destructive as it comes in contact with structures and other molecules within the cell. Without sufficient antioxidants—the natural enemy of free radicals—an excess of free radicals creates inflammation and leads to premature aging. Vitamin C, vitamin E, folate, selenium, and alpha- and beta-carotene, as well as various other phytochemicals, have antioxidant effects.

The vast majority of antioxidants are made available to the body through our consumption of fruit, vegetables, and other natural plants. They are not found in any significant quantity in animal products, nor are they in processed foods. (Phytochemicals have a broad array of beneficial effects outside of their antioxidant role, and these effects are still being studied and need to be further understood.)

Oxidative damage occurs when free-radical activity in cells increases and free radicals burst out of their cellular compartments to affect broader regions of the cell. Free radicals are not all bad; in fact, they have an important role: they chew up waste and can be used by immune cells as they attack and remove damaged cells that could be a danger to us if they continued to deteriorate and potentially developed into cancer. However, the problem with free radicals and other toxins in the cells is that without a relatively robust daily exposure to a broad array of antioxidants and phytochemicals, such as nature intended us to have, the free radicals increase in amount and leave their confined areas. They begin to destroy normal tissue, not just garbage and abnormal tissue. This damages the cells and increases the concentration of cellular toxins.

Because vegetables are so rich in these beneficial compounds, vegetable consumption, especially green vegetable consumption, is an easy way to measure the total antioxidant capacity of a diet. One way scientists can assess our vegetable consumption is with a blood test for alpha-carotene. Beta-carotene, high in carrots and other orange vegetables, is the most widely studied carotenoid, but alpha-carotene more accurately reflects vegetable intake—first because alpha-carotene is not present in most multivitamins and supplements, and second because it is an excellent marker of high-nutrient vegetable intake (given that dark green and orange-colored vegetables are the richest sources of alpha-carotene). Alpha-carotene is one of over forty carotenoids, a family of antioxidants with documented disease-protective and lifespan-promoting benefits.

A recent study measured alpha-carotene in all study participants and then tracked deaths over a fourteen-year follow-up period. The researchers found that increased alpha-carotene was associated with decreased risk of death from all causes. Those with the highest alpha-carotene had a 39 percent decrease in risk of death compared to those with the lowest alpha-carotene.[2] Similar relationships were found between alpha-carotene and risk of death from specific causes—and not just cardiovascular disease and cancer, but other causes as well, notably infection.

Alpha-carotene itself does provide significant antioxidant benefit—but, more important, alpha-carotene is a marker of the thousands of additional compounds in green and orange vegetables, working synergistically to keep the body healthy. Green vegetables are the highest in overall nutrient density, meaning that they contain the most micronutrients per calorie, and of course they are the foods richest in alpha-carotene.

The large, long-term study cited above gives much support to my recommended high-nutrient diet-style, given that many foods high in alpha-carotene tend to be high in other micronutrients overall. When dietary intake of micronutrients (abundant in both diversity and amount) is optimized, a dramatic reduction in later life disease and enhancements in lifespan are possible. In other words, when we eat a significant and diverse amount of unprocessed vegetables, our chances of staying healthier and living longer increase.

Foods with a high ratio of alpha-carotene to calories include the following:

Bok choy	Asparagus
Cabbage	Collards
Red peppers	Broccoli
Carrots	Peas
Swiss chard	Winter squash
Green peppers	

A phytochemically deficient diet is largely responsible for a weak immune system. Populations with a much higher intake of vegetables have much lower rates of cancer, and the longest-living populations throughout history have been those with the highest intake of vegetables in the diet.[3]

I would go so far as to say that phytochemicals are the most important discovery in human nutrition over the last fifty years. Several hundred phytochemical plant nutrients have been identified and about 150 have been studied in detail, though there may be more than a thousand plant-derived molecules that support human immune defenses. The concentration of phytochemicals is often highlighted by vibrant colors of black, blue, red, green, and orange. The classes of phytochemicals contain widely varied structures and unique health benefits, which is why a broad variety is most beneficial.

The variety of types include the following, some of which were introduced above: allium compounds, allyl sulfides, anthocyanins, betalains, coumestans, flavonoids, flavonols glucosinolates, indoles, isoflavones, lignans, liminoids, organosulfides, pectins, phenolic compounds, phytoesterols, protein inhibitors, terpenes (isoprenoids), and tyrosol esters; and there are hundreds of compounds within each category.

Many phytochemicals in freshly harvested plant foods are lost or destroyed by modern processing techniques, including cooking (in some instances). Natural plant foods are highly complex, so their exact structure and the majority of beneficial compounds they contain are still not completely identified. It's clear, though, that the function and production of immune cells are supported by a wide exposure to an assortment of phytochemicals. The lack of a wide assortment of plant-derived phytochemicals in their native form is responsible for the development of most preventable diseases, including cancer.[4]

Just to make this clear, I am saying here that a piece of chicken is like a cookie: they are both foods without a significant antioxidant or phytochemical load. Both animal products and processed foods lack these immunity-supporting nutrients. The more phytochemically deficient foods we eat, the weaker our immunity and the higher our risk of getting sick and possibly developing cancer. The various low-fat diet trends of egg whites, white meats, and pasta are actually immune system–destructive and cancer-causing for various reasons, primarily because of the aforementioned lack of protective phytochemicals.

In various studies, phytochemicals have been found to play protective roles not covered by vitamins and minerals, including the following:

- Inducing detoxification enzymes
- Controlling the production of free radicals
- Deactivating and detoxifying cancer-causing agents
- Protecting cell structures from damage by toxins
- Fueling mechanisms to repair damaged DNA sequences
- Impeding the replication of cells with DNA damage
- Inducing beneficial antifungal, antibacterial, and antiviral effects
- Inhibiting the function of damaged or genetically altered DNA
- Improving immune cells' cytotoxic (destructive) power—that is, the power to kill microbes and cancer cells

This list could be condensed into one primary role: phytochemicals are the fuel that runs our body's anticancer defenses. A diet rich in phytochemicals is the best artillery we have to fight the war on cancer. This defense includes the cell-killing power of the immune system, which needs to be able to destroy invading microbes (viruses and bacteria) and to kill the body's own abnormal cells before they can become cancerous. As DNA "breakages" increase in number, and the cell becomes more and more bizarre, the immune system responds and attempts to remove it. The process of inducing one of the body's abnormal (that is, precancerous or cancerous) cells to die before it can cause damage is called "apoptosis."

Nutrition's Scientific Credentials

Superior nutrition and its impact on human health continues to generate considerable debate and even skepticism, especially as individuals look to defend their prior opinions or dietary preferences. Nevertheless, the vast amount of scientific data demonstrating benefits to immune function—that is, to increasing one's defenses against both infection and cancer—has become overwhelming in recent years.

Any person studying the subject of nutrition in depth and following the latest research would find it hard to ignore the fact that certain natural foods—those that I call "super foods" because they lead to Super Immunity—contain micronutrients that have profound protective effects. The evidence has become overwhelming that devising dietary patterns rich in these high-micronutrient super foods is your secret to excellent health and your access to the fountain of youth.

In the 1930s scientists identified the first known micronutrients: vitamins and minerals. They also isolated the portions of plants that supply us with fuel in the form of calories, labeling those "macronutrients." Macronutrients encompass fat, carbohydrate, and protein. These all contain calories, and we need them to survive. Water is also considered a macronutrient, even though it does not contain calories.

In that same era scientists discovered that a deficiency of certain micronutrients could cause various acute diseases with exotic names like

MACRONUTRIENTS	MICRONUTRIENTS
Fat	Vitamins
Carbohydrate	Minerals
Protein	Phytochemicals
Water	Enzymes

scurvy, pellagra, and beriberi. Deficiency diseases were common in the United States until the 1940s, when the FDA mandated "fortification" (the adding of micronutrients) of common foods like bread and milk. These diseases are still common in many poorer countries, however.

Deficiency of vitamin A—xerophthalmia (an eye disease)
Deficiency of vitamin C—scurvy
Deficiency of vitamin D—rickets and osteoporosis
Deficiency of iodine—goiter and cretinism
Deficiency of iron—anemia and mental retardation
Deficiency of thiamine (B_1)—beriberi
Deficiency of niacin (B_3)—pellagra

By 1940 the vitamin supplement business was a billion-dollar industry: people were advised to drink orange juice and take vitamin C capsules, and our food manufacturers began adding supplemental A, D, and B vitamins to processed foods. In the 1950s and 1960s there was a further increase in fortified processed foods. Eventually processed foods replaced fresh foods as the major source of calories in developed countries.

In the 1960s fast-food restaurants also began to spread throughout America, and by the 1970s they were a six-billion-dollar industry. Within twenty more years they were *everywhere:* in 2005 the fast-food industry broke $120 billion in sales in the United States alone.[5] Fortification of foods became a strategy to prevent deficiency in processed foods that were naturally deficient in micronutrients. Calorie-dense food was everywhere, but the micronutrients were missing. The result? Today, too many of us live on processed foods, convenience foods, and fast foods; we have almost no vegetation, mushrooms, beans, or seeds in our diet.

The fortification of processed foods grew out of an earlier, compartmentalized view of nutritional science: scientists and public authorities thought that we could prevent health complications from poor nutrition, poor food choices, or an inadequate food supply simply by supplying individual micronutrients that were inadequate in the diet. Even though the replacement of these missing nutrients *did* cure and prevent various deficiency diseases (like the ones previously listed), this approach launched a processed-food and junk-food revolution that took our diet and health in the wrong direction.

The mindset that created a shift in our general diet still exists today, and it is still causing damage. These dietary changes not only degraded our immune systems; in the process they exposed us to hundreds of potential illnesses. The oversimplification of human nutrition led to the development of medical foods such as baby formula, hospital liquid feeds, nutritional fortified drinks, and food supplements, further contributing to our health care crisis and ultimately to the explosion of cancer.

The Cancer Explosion in the Modern World

Between 1935 and 2005, cancer rates rose every single year for seventy years straight! As processed foods and fast foods expanded into the underdeveloped world (both nationally and abroad), we saw rural areas starting to develop higher rates of cancer and obesity. The result today is a nation (and other nations) with exploding numbers of people with immune system disorders, allergies, autoimmune diseases, and cancers.

In the 1960s and 1970s most nutritionists focused their attention on the study of macronutrients and looked to determine the best ratio

AVERAGED CANCER MORTALITY TREND
IN THIRTEEN MODERN COUNTRIES

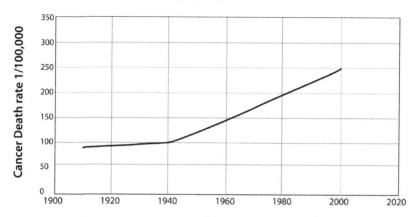

O. Hallberg and O. Johansson, "Cancer Trends During the 20th Century, *Journal of Australian College of Nutritional and Environmental Medicine* 2002, 21(1): 3–8.

of fat, protein, and carbohydrate for optimal health. Doctors and nutritionists thought that our micronutrient needs could be met via a multivitamin or other supplement solution, and saw no necessity to meet our vitamin and mineral needs through micronutrient-rich food. In fact, the micronutrient density of food was generally ignored: science had not yet isolated and understood the critical function and dependence of the immune system on foods that contained hundreds of not-yet-identified organic compounds.

Even today many still believe proper nutrition to be some ideal ratio of macronutrients, with proponents falling into different camps—high-protein advocates, low-fat advocates, high-carb advocates, low-carb advocates, and so on. Unfortunately, this focus on macronutrients over micronutrients diverts attention away from understanding optimal nutrition in a complete and effective manner. Many people worry about their weight, but almost everybody—even the person who carefully monitors caloric intake—neglects their health.

We now know that a diet can be "healthy"—in other words, health-promoting—with a broad range of acceptable macronutrients: it can, for example, contain more fat and less carbohydrate, or more carb and less fat. The problem is that the health-enhancing qualities of a diet are not accurately determined by the level of either fat or carbohydrate. They are determined by the amount and the diversity of micronutrients. For example, a diet with 15 percent fat could be micronutrient-adequate or micronutrient deficient, as could a diet of 40 percent fat. This is a critical point, so I'll restate it: it's not the ratio of fat to carbs in your diet that matters for your health. Many people see fat as the villain and mistakenly ignore the impact of protective micronutrients. They might be surprised to discover that nutritionists have recently learned that when there is fat present in the meal, the most powerful micronutrients found in vegetables are absorbed more readily into the body. In other words, fat itself is not the villain.

The point here is that when our body is deficient in plant-derived micronutrients, we weaken our immune system and leave ourselves exposed to infections and cancer. The way we're going—eating more processed and packaged convenience foods and routinely giving fast food to children—I worry especially about the potential spike in breast cancer rates in younger women in the next twenty to thirty years (or sooner).

I hope that together we can make known the broad array of powerful immune-supporting micronutrients found in vegetables and the incredible opportunity they provide to protect ourselves and our families. The answer is simple—we just need to feed our bodies with super-charged fuel, and that means foods that are richest in micronutrients.

Greens: The King of Vegetables

As we have seen, micronutrients are those nutritional factors essential for our survival and longevity that do not contain calories. Because they are not calorie-contributors, they do not give us fuel or energy;

we rely on *macro*nutrients for that function. The key to superior nutrition, then, is to get adequate amount of micronutrients, while at the same time not consuming excess calories. To get optimal amounts of immune-protective micronutrients, we have to eat lots of vegetables. Fortunately, vegetables are relatively low in calories, so large amounts can be consumed without overeating on calories.

Nutrition scientists have shown over and over that people who eat more natural plant foods—vegetables, fruits, legumes—are less likely to get sick. But are all vegetables equally protective? If we wanted to design a Super Immunity diet, we would want to know which foods had the most powerful effects. Then we could eat plenty of these foods each day, flooding our bodies with the protective substances contained within them.

So . . . which foods have the most powerful effects? Let's add up the immune-supporting micronutrients in a broad array of common foods and see how various food types compare. Later, in chapter 5, I'll give you a similar list for the Top 25 Super Foods.

As you can see from these nutrient scores, when it comes to immune system–building micronutrients, green vegetables win the race. No wonder those are the foods most closely linked with protection against heart disease and cancer. A review of more than 206 epidemiological studies shows that the consumption of raw green vegetables has the most consistent and powerful association with reduction of cancer of all types, including stomach, pancreas, colon, and breast.[6] How many green vegetables do *you* eat a day?

A Matter of *Emphasis*

Most health authorities today are in agreement that we should add more servings of healthy fruits and vegetables to our diet. I disagree. Thinking about our diet in this fashion doesn't adequately address the problem. Instead of considering adding protective fruits, vegetables,

DR. FUHRMAN'S AGGREGATE NUTRIENT DENSITY INDEX (ANDI) SCORES

Kale.................1000	Raspberries............133	Oatmeal 36
Watercress 1000	Blueberries............132	Salmon.................34
Collards 1000	Iceberg lettuce 127	Milk, 1% 31
Swiss chard........... 895	Pomegranates/	Eggs 31
Bok choy 865	pomegranate juice.....119	Bananas................ 30
Spinach 707	Grapes 119	Walnuts............... 30
Arugula 604	Cantaloupe............118	Whole-wheat bread ... 30
Romaine lettuce.......510	Onions............... 109	Almonds 28
Brussels sprouts 490	Plums................ 106	Avocados...............28
Carrots/carrot juice ... 458	Oranges............... 98	White potato...........28
Cabbage 434	Cucumbers.............87	Cashews 27
Broccoli 340	Tofu...................82	Chicken breast.........24
Cauliflower............ 315	Beans (all varieties) 71	Ground beef
Red bell peppers...... 265	Seeds: flax, sunflower,	(85 % lean) 21
Mushrooms 238	sesame, hemp, chia (avg)68	White bread...........17
Asparagus............ 205	Green peas 63	White pasta............16
Tomatoes 186	Cherries................55	Low-fat cheddar cheese. 11
Strawberries..........182	Apples 53	Olive oil 10
Blackberries 171	Peanut butter 51	Corn chips...............7
Leeks.................135	Corn 45	Cola....................1
	Pistachio nuts 37	

To determine the ANDI scores, an equal-calorie serving of each food was evaluated. The following nutrients were included in the evaluation: fiber, calcium, iron, magnesium, phosphorus, potassium, zinc, copper, manganese, selenium, vitamin A, beta carotene, alpha carotene, lycopene, lutein and zeaxanthin, vitamin E, vitamin C, thiamin, riboflavin, niacin, pantothenic acid, vitamin B6, folate, vitamin B12, choline, vitamin K, phytosterols, glucosinolates, angiogenesis inhibitors, organosulfides, aromatase inhibitors, resistant starch, resveratrol plus ORAC score. ORAC (Oxygen Radical Absorbance Capacity) is a measure of the antioxidant or radical scavenging capacity of a food. For consistency, nutrient quantities were converted from their typical measurement conventions (mg, mcg, IU) to a percentage of their Dietary Reference Intake (DRI). For nutrients that have no DRI, goals were established based on available research and current understanding of the benefits of these factors.

To make it easier to compare foods, the raw point totals were converted (multiplied by the same number) so that the highest-ranking foods (leafy green vegetables such as mustard greens, kale and collards) received a score of 1000, and the other foods received lower scores accordingly.

28

beans, seeds, and nuts to our disease-causing diet, *we must make these foods the main focus of the diet itself.*

Once we understand this major mindset-shift and begin to build our diet around fruits, vegetables, beans, seeds, and nuts, *then* we can add foods that are not in this category to the diet.

DR. FUHRMAN'S FOOD PYRAMID

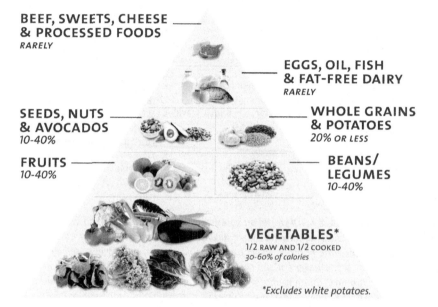

BEEF, SWEETS, CHEESE ____ & PROCESSED FOODS
RARELY

EGGS, OIL, FISH & FAT-FREE DAIRY
RARELY

SEEDS, NUTS & AVOCADOS
10-40%

WHOLE GRAINS & POTATOES
20% OR LESS

FRUITS
10-40%

BEANS/ LEGUMES
10-40%

VEGETABLES*
1/2 RAW AND 1/2 COOKED
30-60% of calories

*Excludes white potatoes.

In a food pyramid, the foods that are consumed in the highest quantity are placed at the base. However, the traditional American food pyramid—the source of most Americans' first understanding of health and nutrition—doesn't put nutrient-rich foods at its base; it gives that place of honor to the bread, cereal, rice, and pasta group. This is one reason why so many Americans are confused about nutrition and plagued by obesity and preventable diseases. Don't you think it makes logical sense to put the healthiest, most micronutrient-rich foods at the base of our food pyramid? Shouldn't we eat more healthy food and less unhealthy food?

My food pyramid is designed to achieve a healthy population. If adopted broadly, it would save millions of people's lives each year and end our costly and tragic health care crisis. There's no way around it: for superior health, we must eat more nutrient-rich foods and fewer calorie-rich foods. Therefore, the top of the pyramid, the foods that should be consumed rarely, contains the foods lowest in nutrients—processed foods like chips and cookies—while the bottom gives a foundation of micronutrient-rich foods. When the nutritional landscape of America is reshaped by nutrient density as represented in the pyramid above, we will radically extend our healthy life expectancy.

Simply put, this means we need to eat lots of high-nutrient, natural plant foods: vegetables, fruits, beans, nuts, and seeds. In conjunction, we need to eat much less from the animal products category and eat far fewer (or no) foods that are completely empty of nutrients or indeed are toxic for the body—foods such as sugar, other sweeteners, white flour, processed foods, refined oils, and fast foods.

Your Remarkable Immune System

It's time to think differently about what we eat and begin to trust the amazing healing and protective power of the body.

It's time for all of us to reconsider the notion that viruses are the sole or even the primary cause of serious viral-associated illnesses. Most often the exposure to and presence of a virus, and its association with the disease and its complications, is *not* the only cause and not even the *main* cause that initiates an illness. Certainly, exposure to the virus and its multiplication within our body is at the core of viral infections. However, though it is not generally recognized, the virus adapts itself to the host (our body) and becomes dangerous and multiplies *as a result of the host's disease-promoting environment,* created by nutritional inadequacy. In most cases, a virus, when exposed to a healthy, well-nourished body, would remain harmless. Our vulnerability to the initial virus and our inability to fight off the virus once we have become exposed is directly affected by the quality of our diet prior to being exposed. This means that poor nutrition not only makes us more susceptible to viruses but significantly impacts the length and severity of an illness.

Poor nutrition is so ubiquitous that we can consider 98 percent of Americans to be at significant disease risk. This, coupled with the enhanced resistance of bacteria from the use and overuse of antibiotics, has created a new era in modern health science with dangerous antibiotic-resistant diseases exploding. Deaths from infectious diseases increased by 58 percent between 1980 and 1992 in the United States, and the figure has continued to increase since then. According to Hiroshi Nakajima, director-general of the World Health Organization in the decade 1988–1998, "We are standing on the brink of a global crisis in infectious diseases."[7]

Traditionally, the etiology (or cause) of infections, both bacterial and viral, has the following elements. These are the primary factors that determine whether you get sick or not; and when you do get sick, how sick you get.

1. *The size of the inoculum.* In other words, how much of the virus or bacterium was present in the exposure?

2. *The virulence of the exposure.* How powerful a disease-causing agent was that microbe?

3. *The immune-response of the host.* Was there an opportunity for the host's immune memory to that microbe (or a similar microbe) to facilitate a rapid and potentially protective immune response; could the immune system quickly remove the virus before it replicated itself in large numbers?

4. *The nutritional status and health of the host.* Was the host's immune-competency compromised, or could the immune system react to

its full potential in inhibiting and eventually subduing the viral invasion of normal cells?

For the most part we don't have the opportunity to modify these risk factors substantially, though with handwashing and other proper hygienic measures, such as not touching our own face without washing first, we can diminish some of the exposure risks. However, there is one major factor well within our control that can alter the equation. That is, we can maintain comprehensive nutritional adequacy (CNA). Comprehensive nutritional adequacy means that a sufficient amount and variety of all known and unknown micronutrients are present. Very few of us currently have CNA because our present dietary model contains too many processed foods that are micronutrient-barren. For most of us to achieve CNA, we need to change our diet and begin to eat all of the immune-supporting nutrients available to us.

Think about what I'm saying: a viral exposure that would cause a serious or even life-threatening infection in a person eating the conventional diet would not even result in symptoms of illness in a nutritionally competent person. Let's stop here for a moment and revisit the implications of this. We now have scientific evidence that clearly demonstrates the dangers of nutritional incompetency. And yet far too many of us still aren't aware of the essential nutritional factors that support and sustain our everyday health. Together, we can change this.

We often hear comments such as "The virus attacked his heart" or "She had a virally induced cancer," and yet we rarely consider or address the issues that enabled the virulence of that virus. We aren't just targets waiting to be attacked; in fact, a healthy body is highly resistant to viral attack. It has already been demonstrated that when children eat more vegetables, they have fewer infections. A study on relatively malnourished children in Vietnam illustrated this. Young children (five months to two years old) were randomly selected and assigned based on local areas to one of two groups, *nutritional intervention* or *control*. The intervention group received more vegetables and other micronutrient-rich food, while the control group was left on the typical rice diet. During follow-up, children in the intervention communes had approximately half the respiratory illness experienced by those in comparison communes.[8] It is now accepted in scientific circles that micronutrient deficiencies contribute to the mortality and morbidity of infectious diseases, and that a more micronutrient-rich diet is needed for better human health.[9]

The Dangers of Virus Mutation

The relationship between nutritional status and the immune system has been a topic of study for over fifty years, as we have seen. In the last twenty years a much greater understanding of the complexity of the immune response and its dependence on nutritional factors has evolved. Dramatic increases in our understanding of the immune system and the nutritional factors that regulate immune function have demonstrated a remarkable concordance between host nutritional status and immunity to almost all known infectious agents.[10]

There are two main points here that we will explore further:

1. The nutritional status of the host is critical in permitting or preventing viral and bacterial infections.

2. Nutritional inadequacies in the host allow the modification of viruses into more virulent or dangerous forms.

The concept that powerful and competent host defenses are enabled by nutritional excellence is not just an opinion or observation; it is the reality of human physiology supported by hundreds of scientific studies. When the body is deprived of nutrients, viral infections can cause serious, even fatal diseases that don't occur when deficiency is not present.[11] Immunity, when optimized, can ward off infection; and if infection does occur, it is much more likely to have a harmless outcome.

When discussing interactions of nutrition and infection, nutritionists have traditionally considered only the effects of diet on the host (us). It has been known for years that malnutrition interferes with various physical barriers or immune responses, making the body more vulnerable to attack from microbes, including viruses. Newer evidence is now showing that the level of nutrition of the host can also directly influence the genetic makeup of the virus, altering its virulence.[12] In other words, excellent nutrition can both indirectly and directly promote resistance to infectious disease.

The most effective artillery we have to protect ourselves against the potentially damaging effects of influenza and other infectious disease is nutritional excellence. *And that's in our own, individual control!*

If you are deficient in virtually any known vitamin or mineral, research has shown that your defense functions can be negatively affected. Most notably, it has been demonstrated that when diets are low in consumption of green and yellow vegetables (rich in carotenoids), viral illnesses takes a more serious form. Multiple micronutrients, including lutein, lycopene, folate, bioflavonoids, riboflavin, zinc, selenium, and many others have immune-modulating functions.[13] We will learn much more about these later. But what it comes down to is this: their presence or absence strengthens or weakens the ability of the immune system, influencing our susceptibility to infectious diseases and the course and outcome of such diseases.

The ability of the nutritionally competent immune system to prevent viral genetic mutations that would allow the virus to evade the host's defenses has been recognized in varying investigations, even those studying HIV (human immunodeficiency virus).[14] Micronutrient deficiencies are prevalent in many HIV-infected populations, and numerous studies have reported that these deficiencies impair immune responses and are associated with accelerated HIV disease progression.

For example, numerous studies have demonstrated that the transmission of the AIDS virus is significantly reduced (and even made improbable) when the host's nutrition is excellent. This means that eating a micronutrient-rich diet, with no notable deficiencies, may be the most critical factor in our ability, individually, to combat emerging infections; with the weapon of good nutrition, we enable our body to have control over viral replication inside us and prohibit the virus from transforming to evade capture.[15] Viral replication accompanied by changes in the virus as it replicates enables the virus to hide from our immune system surveillance and control. However, these dangerous structural modifications to the virus as it replicates occur only in a nutritionally incompetent host.

More recently, research has shown that the influenza virus also exhibits increased virulence in a nutritionally deficient host, allowing multiple changes in the viral genome. In other words, your everyday flu can mutate and become able to cause more serious damage to the lungs and other parts of the body. Although it has been known for many years that poor nutrition can affect host response to infection, the finding that host nutrition also affects the genetic sequence of a pathogen (a disease-causing microbe) is recent—an important finding for us now and as a field of future investigation.

A good example is a recent scientific study that investigated the nutritional status of patients who developed neuropathy (nerve damage) after a viral illness. Those people whose nervous system was damaged by the virus were found to be deficient in riboflavin, vitamin E, selenium, alpha- and beta-carotenes, and lycopene. When patients were supplemented with these nutrients, the disease began to subside, suggesting that the pathogenicity of a particular virus—that is, the ability of a pathogen to produce an infectious disease—is dependent on the nutritional status of the host.[16]

As the data suggests, a nutritarian diet is an effective intervention for viral diseases such as HIV, mononucleosis, herpes, and influenza, because viral mutations will be suppressed, limiting disease-causing potential and virulence.

Unfortunately, most of the food that the majority of Americans consume weakens rather than strengthens their normal resistance to simple viral infections. Despite advances in science that have revealed the critical importance of thousands of protective micronutrients in the natural plant kingdom, much of the modern world consumes a diet rich in processed grains, oils, sweets, and animal products. In the United States, for example, less than 5 percent of total calories consumed come from fresh fruits, vegetables, seeds, and nuts. And yet these are the foods that are richest in micronutrients!

Those who eat the standard American diet, with an overabundance of calories but a very low nutrient-per-calorie intake, are in a chronically malnourished condition. This combination of being overweight yet malnourished is the true life-threatening epidemic in the modern world, resulting in a medical care crisis and avoidable medical tragedies. With the ubiquitous consumption of low-nutrient processed foods, nutritional deficiency has become the norm.

The global demographic impact of the 1918–19 influenza pandemic continues to fascinate researchers and scholars. When we look into the effects of this outbreak on society, through a comprehensive investigation of the modes of transmission and propagation, mortality rates, and distinctive features of various regions, we see the importance of taking a country's unique stresses and nutritional habits into account. For example, Iran was one of the regions hit hardest by the pandemic, with mortality rates significantly higher than in most regions of the world. The research suggests that famine, opium, malaria, and anemia were fundamentally responsible for the high flu mortality in that country. Those with compromised immunity suffered the most damage.[17] As it is today, the diet in western Europe in those days was largely meat, bread, potato, lard, butter, and cheese, with minimal fresh produce. However, this occurred during World War I and almost 2 percent of those infected died from a secondary infection: bacterial pneumonia. It affected many young soldiers because the close troop quarters, the stresses of combat and war, and their malnourished state all contributed to their depressed immune system function, increasing their susceptibility.

In the past, scientists focused on the effects of nutritional deficiencies on the people themselves, never on the invading microbes. Now we know that increasingly dangerous microbes are created inside a nutrient-deficient host—and the diets of yore were grossly deficient. Without the knowledge of the need for vitamin C, a multitude of micronutrients in fresh greens, and vitamin D from the sun—all of these difficult to procure in the past during the winter, when produce and sunshine were scarce—viral epidemics were common.

The association between famine and epidemics has been noted throughout human history. And yet, despite the fact that we have new science pointing to impressive nutritional disease protection against heart disease, strokes, dementia, cancer, and yes, serious infections, we still consume a diet assuring nutritional compromise and resulting in tragic medical outcomes.

It's time for us to get off our chicken and pasta low-fat diets or our cheeseburgers and Cokes. We need to get our heads out of the french fries and begin to change the way we think about what we eat and its impact on our health. The link between superior nutrition and Super Immunity is an opportunity—a privilege to apply and share. Science shows us the protection offered by immune-strengthening compounds found in cruciferous vegetables, raw vegetables, beans, fruits, nuts, and seeds. We *all* have the amazing potential to live a long, healthy life with Super Immunity. The epidemiological studies, the controlled research studies, and the clinical experience have put forth a preponderance of evidence that is now overwhelming and should be impossible to ignore. This is not *alternative* medicine; it is *progressive* medicine, it is *good* medicine.

CHAPTER TWO

The Failure of
Modern Medicine

My husband and I have three children, all of whom have been following Dr. Fuhrman's nutritional guidance since birth. None of them has had any major illness. On the rare occasion that they have a fever (my six-year-old has had about three fevers in his life, my four-year-old has had only one, and my sixteen-month-old has never had one), it lasts for the afternoon and is gone by the time they wake up from their nap or by the time they get up in the morning. We don't use fever-reducing medication. We do not vaccinate against the flu. None of my children has ever had the flu. When friends and cousins around them are sick and coughing, our children do not succumb. Illness that can linger in other children for weeks at a time (both my husband's sister's children and my sister's children are often sick for days or weeks at a time) passes over our children completely.

—Diana Ricci

Very high mortality rates prevailed in Europe throughout medieval times. This was a result of both deficiencies in sanitation and insufficient food for a population that had expanded faster than agriculture. Mortality rates were further complicated by frequent warfare and exploitation of civilians by brutal rulers. Life for the average person at that time was stressful and often short.

However, there have been areas around the world and throughout history where relatively healthy diets and peaceful environments encouraged long and healthy lives. For example, the Hunzas in the Himalayas, Peruvian natives living in the Andes, and the Okinawans of northern Japan all had average lifespans well exceeding modern averages.

The main reasons for premature deaths in earlier centuries were violence and infection. Infectious diseases decreased markedly in the last few hundred years, mostly as the result of the availability of clean water and, in the last century, flush toilets to eliminate waste. A dramatic decline in most infections occurred as our sanitation practices were improved in cities and standardized across the modern world.[1] This decline in infectious disease due to plumbing (not medical advances!) is the main factor accounting for the overall increases in lifespan that is claimed in modern times.

However, it remains unclear whether adults are actually living longer than they did in prior centuries. Certainly the *average* lifespan of adults has increased, mostly because fewer infants and toddlers are now dying of infections, and fewer women are dying in childbirth. That said, lifespan advances in adult males (that is, non–childbirth related) have not improved significantly, because reductions in later-life, infectious-disease related deaths were more than compensated for by increases in chronic diseases of nutritional ignorance and dietary excess. As processed foods, fast foods, and commercially mass-produced animal products became the dietary norm, heart disease, strokes, and cancer increased to fill the void left by the decreased impact of infectious diseases.

In fact, to counter the common argument that we are living longer compared to earlier times, consider that we have good records on the lifespan achieved by over 150 male Renaissance artists living in the fourteenth century, whose average age of death was considerably higher than that of the average male in America today.[2] Advancements in medicine and pharmacology are largely credited for major advances in health and in saving lives. But the reality is this: medical care has little effect on the overall health quality or even the average age of death in modern societies worldwide.

If fact, exposure to medical care and resources spent on health care are linked to *decreases* in healthy life expectancy, not increases.[3] Emergency medical care is valuable, but in the modern world emergencies linked to injury, accidents, and infection are no longer the leading causes of death. Heart disease, strokes, and cancer are now the big three.

Treating bad nutritional choices with drugs—choices that lead to morbidity in later life, after years and years of self-abuse—will never be an efficacious solution.

Most of what doctors do to treat today's diseases does little to extend human lifespan; in the majority of cases, it is almost worthless. Why so? Because the drugs prescribed by doctors encourage patients' risky lifestyle behaviors and self-destructive eating choices to continue; they give patients "permission" to continue poor behaviors because they mask the symptoms of disease. The symptoms are not the actual pathology (or damage); they are just markers that the pathology has developed. Treating the symptoms does not halt the advancing pathology, which in all likelihood will continue to worsen. That "solution" is akin to your mechanic's "fixing" the flashing oil light on your car's dashboard by simply snipping the wire to the light. If today's symptom-suppressing medications were not available, more effective lifestyle modifications could be insisted on by physicians and advisors in authority and thus would more likely be implemented by their patients and the general population.

When considering the risks of any medication or medical intervention, we have to also consider the benefits of lifestyle interventions, such as salt avoidance, exercise, dietary modifications, and weight reduction—interventions that have no side effects and whose focus is on removing the cause, not just treating the symptoms.

Medications in Candyland

John Abramson, M.D., clinical professor at Harvard and author of *Overdosed America*, explains that we have to consider the context when reviewing any medical intervention, because the information doctors receive about medical interventions is heavily biased toward intervention and treatment. The studies are funded and the results interpreted by the pharmaceutical companies, or at least influenced by their funding sponsors. What is published in the most prestigious medical journals is no longer careful science, but essentially drug advertisements. The information brought to and taught to the medical profession is shaped by its commercial value to the drug companies, and the fundamental purpose is to improve corporate profits.

Modern medical care evolved as a drug-distribution arm of the pharmaceutical industry, not a profession concerned primarily with improving people's health. A true health care system focused on maximizing patients' well-being would center around removing impediments to better health, promotion of healthy habits (such as smoking cessation, exercise, and dietary improvement), and protection against exposure to chemicals, toxins, and other known causes of disease. Instead, prescription drugs, which all have toxicities and dangers, have become the primary intervention for every dietary-induced health issue.

For example, consider the effectiveness of a handful of the most popular drugs prescribed for the lowering of blood pressure or blood sugar in diabetics. A recent study of over 90,000 type 2 diabetics compared the cardiovascular effects in individuals treated with either metformin or a sulfonylurea-class drug—two of the most popular drugs. Similar to the outcomes of earlier studies, researchers found an increased likelihood of death, averaging about 40 percent in the patients treated with sulfonylureas, and also about a 25 percent increased risk of congestive heart failure.[4]

Simply put, lowering blood glucose with medications does not remove the causes of type 2 diabetes—physical inactivity and excess weight from a calorie-rich, nutrient-poor diet. Excess body fat blocks insulin function and forces the pancreas to overproduce insulin. Over time, the overworked pancreas "poops out." Giving drugs to force the already overworked and failing pancreas to work even harder only makes the insulin-producing cells die off faster. If you are still eating the same disease-causing diet, you will likely gain *more* weight, develop *more* cardiovascular disease, and eventually become insulin-dependent.

Medication has become the accepted treatment for diabetes—even though the medications themselves often promote weight gain and increased appetite and can make the individual more diabetic. These medications also significantly increase the incidence of cancer at multiple sites.[5] In addition to all these side effects, controlling blood glucose with drugs has *not* been shown to decrease the risk of death—in fact, it increases risk. The ACCORD (Action to Control Cardiovascular Risk in Diabetes) study was conducted to determine whether lowering glucose to near-normal levels with drugs would decrease cardiovascular risk; however, the study was halted when the results showed that more medications to better control blood sugar actually increased the risk of death from all causes and from cardiovascular disease.[6] If you don't address the primary cause—a disease-causing diet—just adding more and more medications is futile.

Contrary to public perception, attempts to lower blood pressure with drugs have similar negative consequences. Consider, for example, angiotensin receptor blockers (ARBs), which are used to treat high blood pressure and heart failure, and are actually one of the safer drug categories available for lowering blood pressure. They work by blocking a hormone system that regulates vascular tone and water and salt balance to control blood pressure. The hormone angiotensin can affect cell survival and angiogenesis (formation of new blood vessels), two important factors in tumor growth. The issue here is the concern that these medications may promote the growth of blood vessels that could enable the growth of tumors and cancers.

To determine whether taking ARBs affects cancer risk, scientists performed a meta-analysis of several studies. They determined that ARBs carry a significantly increased risk of a new diagnosis of any cancer (8 percent) and a seriously higher risk of lung cancer (25 percent).[7] The study also revealed increased rates of sudden cardiac death, death from heart attack, and death from stroke in the subjects taking an ARB compared to those taking placebos in two studies; this data is still being reviewed by the FDA.[8]

Consider another blood pressure drug class: beta-blockers. In the large POISE (Perioperative Ischemic Evaluation) trial, conducted in twenty-three countries, all 8,351 enrolled patients were randomized to either metoprolol (a common beta-blocker) or a placebo. After thirty days, overall mortality (death) was higher in the group treated with the beta-blocker—3.1 percent vs. 2.3 percent—and the drug-treated group had almost double the incidence of stroke.[9] Additional analyses did not identify any subgroup that benefited from metoprolol. The artificially lowered blood pressure had clear risks; the drugs caused more harm than good.

In fact, there is no data to suggest that these drugs prevent heart attacks in healthy people with only mildly elevated blood pressure. The latest review of the evidence was presented in a 2007 issue of the *Journal of the American College of Cardiology*.[10] Despite three decades of physicians using beta-blockers for hypertension, the authors of the state-of-the-art paper noted that no study has shown that beta-blocker therapy reduces death in hypertensive patients, even when compared with placebos. A review conducted by the highly respected Cochrane Database of Systematic Reviews found essentially the same thing: the prescriptions written for beta-blockers to lower blood pressure do not extend lifespan.[11]

The liberal use of medications in an attempt to reduce the effects of our toxic diet-style has its own set of unique risks, as these research findings suggest. Medications to lower blood pressure also cause fatigue, lightheadedness, and loss of balance. They can lead to falls in the elderly, potentially causing hip fractures, and they can lower diastolic blood pressure excessively (as they lower systolic), which increases the potential for cardiac arrhythmias, potentially leading to death.[12] Blood pressure medications that lower diastolic blood pressure too far have also been shown to increase the occurrence of atrial fibrillation, another serious rhythm disturbance of the heart.[13]

In the elderly, moderately high blood pressure is not a risk factor for increased mortality. *Low* blood pressure, on the other hand, is: blood pressure values below 140/70 are associated with excess mortality in the elderly, and this is especially noticeable when drugs push down the diastolic blood pressure too low.[14]

Systolic pressure is the first, higher number; it represents the force of the heart pumping against the resistance offered by the blood vessel walls. Diastolic pressure is the second, lower number; it represents the pressure against the blood vessels during the relaxation and filling phase of the heartbeat. When blood vessels stiffen with disease and aging, the systolic rises because the vessels do not expand during systole as they should, and the diastolic falls because the blood vessel wall no longer contracts inward as it should.

Because coronary artery filling occurs during diastole, people with coronary artery disease (CAD) are at increased risk for coronary ischemic events (caused by insufficient blood flow and oxygenation) when diastolic blood pressure falls below a certain level. This is because when diastolic blood pressure is too low, the heart does not refill adequately with blood during diastole. When international researchers studied 22,000 patients in a fourteen-country study, they found a striking increase in heart attacks in those whose medications brought the diastolic blood pressure below 84. Those with a diastolic blood pressure below 60 had three times the occurrence of heart attacks compared to those with a diastolic above 80! We often have to look outside this country for some balanced research.

Whether it's cold medications, antibiotics, pain medications, immunizations, or blood pressure or diabetic medications, the false perception is that these are life-saving interventions dramatically extending our lives. Our confusion is understandable: generally speaking, drug studies are designed to hide potential side effects, and the long-term negative outcomes from drug use are most often hidden or unknown. The side effects and risks of using *multiple* drugs at the same time are even greater. The dangers of this major health issue are profound, rarely investigated, and impossible to predict. In recent years, more and more emergency room visits and hospital admissions are due to the effects of medications. For example, consider the following limited list:[15]

Drug Class	Emergency Visits	Hospital Admissions
Antibiotics	95,000	131,300
Narcotics	44,300	121,200
Anticoagulants	29,200	218,800
Steroids	13,300	283,700

Our bodies are highly resilient and self-repairing, but medicines cannot enable us to escape the biological laws of cause and effect. When we damage ourselves with exposure to toxic, disease-causing diets, we develop diseases.

Medicines cannot drug away the
cellular defects that develop in response to
improper nutrition throughout life.

The point here is that we have to be responsible for our own health and rely on vigilant avoidance of the underlying causes of disease. We need to adopt scientifically supported superior nutrition and rid ourselves of the idea that doctors and pharmaceutical companies are our saviors, capable of enabling us to live long and productive lives.

The Pros and Cons of Flu Shots

All medical interventions have a benefit-to-risk ratio. Each person has to weigh the supposed benefits against the potential risks. Often the long-term risks of medications are not clearly delineated, however, and most of the time they are not adequately investigated. The supposed benefits are almost always exaggerated by pharmaceutical companies and the authorities in their sphere of influence in medicine and government.

Flu vaccines have benefits and risks as well. Researchers and physicians study these issues and attempt to ascertain if the benefits outweigh the risks, but no scientific person studying this issue would conclude that immunizations are *without* risk. So to consider whether getting vaccinated against the flu is wise and advisable, we have to look at how effective flu shots are and then weigh that against the known (and potential additional unknown) risks. When reviewing this information, keep in mind that the dangers of the flu are highest in sickly and poorly nourished individuals; healthy people have little to fear from the simple flu.

Flu Facts

We are told that about 10 percent of U.S. residents get influenza each year. About 100,000 are hospitalized, and it is most often quoted that 36,000 Americans die from complications of the flu each year. But that is an older statistic that is now questioned. A recent study, in government reports, provides updated estimates of the range of flu-associated deaths that occurred in the United States during the three decades prior to 2007. The CDC estimates that from the 1976–1977 season to the 2006–2007 season, flu-associated deaths ranged from a low of about 3,000 per year to a high of about 49,000. So an average of 25,000 is more accurate.[16] The biggest complication and cause of death in someone with the flu is bacterial pneumonia, which develops most often in elderly or immunosuppressed individuals. The symptoms of the flu include:

- High fever

- Headache

- Extreme fatigue

- Muscle aches

- Cough, sore throat, nasal congestion (common but not universal)

- Gastrointestinal symptoms, such as nausea, vomiting, and diarrhea (more common in children)

Of these symptoms, it is primarily severe headaches and muscle aches that usually differentiate the flu from other viral illnesses (such as colds).

People stay contagious for about a week after contracting the standard flu. The good news is that, if you are generally healthy and eat a healthy diet, consuming a high percentage of your calories from fruits, vegetables, seeds, and nuts, you need not panic. The flu is not a dangerous disease in healthy individuals. Even the more virulent and dangerous flu strains, such as the avian flu, stand little chance against a truly healthy immune system.

Forty percent of Americans die of heart attacks and strokes, but almost all of these deaths are avoidable with excellent nutrition. About 35 percent of all Americans die of cancer; likewise, the vast majority of these deaths are the result of poor nutrition. Indeed, the premise of this book is that today's epidemic of cancer is not predominantly genetic; rather, it is mostly the result of nutritionally handicapped immune systems. When we eat a nutrient-scarce diet, diseases flourish. With nutritional excellence, our body becomes a miraculous, disease-resistant organism. The flu is no exception.

The Purported Benefits of Flu Shots

The issue is not whether the flu can be harmful and even in rare cases cause death; we know it can. The issue is how much of that morbidity and mortality can be reduced by vaccination. The influenza vaccine is frequently cited as a means to reduce morbidity and mortality associated with infection, and the CDC (U.S. Centers for Disease Control and Prevention) now recommends universal influenza vaccination for all individuals starting at age six months or older. But how effective is the vaccination?

For the first time, the CDC's recommendations now include healthy adults who are not in contact with individuals at high risk for the complications of influenza. The recommendation for vaccinating healthy adults is built upon several assumptions:

- The vaccine will reduce the number of cases of influenza.
- The vaccine will reduce complications of influenza.
- The vaccine will reduce the transmission of influenza.
- The vaccine will accomplish these goals *safely*.

Over 200 separate viruses cause the flu and flulike illnesses whose symptoms include fever, cough, headaches, body aches and pains, and a runny nose. Even with the best-case scenario, during years when the most prevalent strains of influenza A and B have been correctly guessed at and included for the following season in the design of the vaccine, the flu shot still covers less than 10 percent of the circulating viruses creating these illnesses. In the real world, the viral strains that are chosen for the vaccine simply cannot be an exact match with those circulating; only a partial match is ever achieved. So how effective is flu vaccine at preventing flu?

Moreover, can the vaccine prevent *complications* of influenza, which occur very rarely among adults without chronic illness? The best way we have to answer these questions is to look at the current analysis from the earlier-cited, highly respected Cochrane Database of Systematic Reviews, which investigates such issues. Cochrane finds weak evidence of vaccine efficacy.[17]

These researchers examined medical databases through June 2010 for randomized, controlled trials of influenza vaccines. Nonrandomized trials were also included if they provided safety data regarding the vaccine. The main study outcome was the number of influenza infections and the seriousness of infection symptoms. Researchers also followed rates of influenza complications and the number of working days lost. Finally, the risk for adverse events associated with the influenza vaccine was evaluated. The review included fifty studies involving over 70,000 participants. Considering how avidly our U.S. health authorities promote the flu vaccine, the findings were surprising: this independent analysis of the data revealed that vaccine use did *not* affect the number of people hospitalized or days lost from work. Furthermore, none of the different influenza vaccines had a significant effect in reducing the risk of complications of influenza among healthy adults.

These investigators also reviewed the risk for serious adverse events associated with the use of the influenza vaccine. The review determined that the vaccine may promote an additional 1.6 cases of Guillain-Barré syndrome for each million vaccinations given. Guillain-Barré syndrome is a nerve disorder that starts as loss of sensation and then progresses to muscle weakness and paralysis, including inability to breathe.

Overall, the review found the evidence for universal vaccination to be underwhelming and were critical of the CDC's recommendations for healthy adults.

The Cochrane review made it clear that about half the trials reviewed were funded by the vaccine companies and observed that, in such cases, the results are questionable, because such trials include only ideal viral-matching conditions and also limit the tracking of harm. Cochrane investigators noted widespread manipulation of the conclusions in such vaccine-manufacturer-funded studies. But even when looking at these biased studies, where the vaccine was well matched to the circulating virus, we see that vaccination against influenza was far from fully protective against infection, that the vaccine did not significantly impact the number of days of work missed, and that it did not prevent complications of influenza.

The Cochrane review also looked specifically at the vaccination of children against the flu. After reviewing the data on fifty-one studies addressing the effectiveness and safety of flu vaccines for children, the Cochrane reviewers were shocked with our government's policy of universal vaccination. They found that in children under the age of two, the effectiveness of the vaccine was similar to that of a placebo. They also found it impossible to analyze the safety of vaccines from the available studies, due to the lack of recorded data in the trials. More concerning was their conclusion that the safety outcome data was not feasible due to extensive evidence of reporting bias in the studies. The Cochrane authors were again critical of the CDC's decisions, stating, "If immunization in children is to be recommended as a public health policy, large-scale studies assessing important outcomes and directly comparing vaccine types are urgently needed."[18]

Even among the elderly, where the risk of death from infections is higher, the studies on flu vaccination are not definitively favorable. A review of influenza vaccination among adults at age sixty-five or older suggested that the vaccine was of questionable efficacy.[19] While vaccination appeared to reduce the symptoms of influenza, the poor quality of the collected research prevented any strong conclusion regarding the effectiveness of the vaccine in preventing complications of influenza, even in this high-risk population.

The fact that flu vaccination is heavily promoted by government and medical authorities, despite the marginal benefits, fuels distrust of the entire medical/pharmaceutical/government health complex, which reeks of collusion and conflict of interest. This situation is reflective of a foundational problem with health care today: governmental authorities shaping our personal medical decisions are heavily influenced by commercial interests wielding political donations, by powerful lobbyists, and by industry-funded experts.

The scientists from the Cochrane Database of Systematic Reviews were quite pointed in their critique of public health efforts in the United States to heavily promote increased usage of the vaccine: "The CDC authors clearly do not weigh interpretation by the quality of the evidence, but quote anything that supports their theory." No wonder, because almost all of the fifteen members of the CDC's Advisory Committee on Immunization Practices have financial ties to the vaccine industry! The CDC grants them waivers from statutory conflict-of-interest rules. Their professional experience contributes to the development of their immunization expertise—at least, that is the rationale offered by the CDC to justify the waivers.[20]

The Known Risks of Flu Shots

If you read about the flu vaccine in the information supplied by the manufacturer, you will learn that each dose contains traces of formaldehyde and 25 micrograms of thimerosal (a mercury-containing compound), the latter used as a preservative. The injection of even this small amount of mercury year after year may place a person at increased risk of neurotoxicity later in life. The actual extent of this risk is hard to ascertain.

We do know that risks accumulate throughout life and that the young, developing body is more sensitized to the damaging effects of toxic substances. The American Academy of Pediatrics and the U.S. Public Health Service, a federal agency, have issued a joint statement calling for the removal of mercury from all vaccines. Chronic, low-dose mercury exposure may cause subtle neurological abnormalities that rear their head later in life. Considering all the vaccines children get already, adding flu vaccine to the mix and giving it each year is something that we should have serious questions about—and indeed, the scientific literature has raised those questions.

If we are going to advise giving a flu shot to everybody from infancy on, every single year, the long-term effects must be more closely examined. The flu vaccine itself has not yet been evaluated for carcinogenic potential, and animal reproductive studies over multiple years have not been performed—in other words, studies in animals testing whether the vaccine causes birth defects or developmental problems or even if it increases the risk of cancer.

Known adverse reactions to the vaccine, according to the manufacturer, include arthralgia (joint pain), lymphadenopathy (swelling of lymph nodes), itching, vasculitis (inflammation of blood vessels), and other events reflective of toxicity. Allergic reactions such as hives and anaphylaxis, neurological disorders such as neuritis, encephalitis, and optic neuritis, and—besides the previously mentioned Guillian-Barré syndrome—demyelenating disorders (such as multiple sclerosis) have also been temporally associated with influenza vaccine. There will likely be more connections made: in the ordinary life cycle of a drug, as time goes on more side effects are typically uncovered. Most recently, influenza vaccinations have been implicated as a trigger for Henoch-Schonlein purpura, a rare but serious disease that can cause kidney failure.[21]

Each person needs to decide the risk-to-benefit ratio for themselves and their own children, because serious complications and even death from a simple viral illness such as the flu *can* occur. Still, with the limited effectiveness of today's vaccines, the benefits, even in high-risk groups, are slight.

The medical community acknowledges that certain people are at greater risk of harm and death from the flu. Those with weakened immune systems are at increased risk when they catch an infection of any type. This group includes:

- The elderly—those over seventy-five
- Those with chronic medical conditions, such as diabetes, transplanted organs, or AIDS
- Steroid-dependent individuals or those on other immunosuppressive drugs for autoimmune illness
- Those with significant immunosuppression (such as people with AIDS or cancer)
- Infants and toddlers under two years of age who were not breast-fed
- Those who smoke cigarettes or whose food intake is primarily junk food and other high-calorie, low-nutrient fast foods or packaged foods

In these groups, the slight reduction in influenza virulence for just a limited number of strains may be of benefit. This is not the case in healthy children or adults with normal immune function, however—especially if people are eating a nutritious diet and have adequate nutritional stores, including vitamin D.

I prefer to feed my children in a manner that protects them against *all* diseases and simply allow their healthy immune systems to deal with the flu, should they get it. My four children, who now range in age from ten to twenty-four, almost never have been sick for more than a few days in their whole lives, never had an ear infection or needed an antibiotic, and never, to my recollection, ever got the flu. Maybe good nutrition had something to do with it.

We should all be appropriately fearful of the flu. Maybe that fear would encourage us to take action and start eating large amounts of nutrient-rich natural foods. Presently we don't, as a nation—but if we did, the fear of the flu could actually save millions of lives, because the same healthy diet that protects against the flu also protects against many cancers, heart disease, diabetes, obesity, asthma, and other diseases.

Other Flu-Related Issues

While flu shots are a hot-button topic these days—and rightfully so, as we have seen—there are other flu-related topics to consider.

More Drug Options for the Flu

When you get the flu, many physicians prescribe drugs that are marketed as helping you get better faster. Three antiviral drugs— amantadine (brand name Symmetrel), rimantadine (Flumadine), and oseltamivir (Tamiflu)—are available in the United States for influenza. These medications are only partially effective, and they are not effective at all unless they are started within the first two days of symptoms. As prescription drugs, they have serious potential risks. Besides the more common side effects of nausea, vomiting, dizziness, and insomnia, rare but serious adverse reactions have been reported, including depression, suicide, and a potentially fatal reaction called neuroleptic malignant syndrome, which involves a high fever, muscle rigidity, and mental status changes.

The general use of these medications has a poor benefit-to-risk ratio, especially since it is hard to differentiate influenza from other, similar viral infections, for which these medications would *not* be indicated. Most prescriptions for these drugs are written without clear documentation of a flu virus being responsible. It takes time to diagnose the flu, and by the time a person gets to a doctor for an accurate diagnosis, the window of time in which these medications are effective will have passed. Hundreds of thousands of doses of Tamiflu are prescribed each year, and in more than 90 percent of instances, they will be used after the period when the drug has any potential to help! People will be increasing their risk of medication-caused side effects *without any potential benefit*.

The poor benefit-to-risk ratio would make it hard for anyone to recommend the general use of these medications. However, these medications may be appropriate in the event of an outbreak in a nursing home or hospital—places where high-risk people are in close contact with one another and an early diagnosis of the flu can be confirmed.

The Protection of Good Hygiene

Almost every year flu season seems to bring with it extraordinary anxiety and fear, especially among parents of young children. Through all the fog of media hysteria and worry, let's not lose our bearing and make rash decisions to use medications that can cause more harm than good.

The important news is that most Americans can and should take steps to reduce the likelihood of getting an infectious disease like the flu. Viruses are primarily spread via hand-to-face contact. They can also be spread when a sick person coughs or sneezes, aerosolizing the virus so others inhale it. A person can be contagious the day before he or she develops symptoms and for seven to ten days after symptoms first develop.

Here are some steps you can take to minimize the likelihood of catching the flu:

Avoid touching your face when you are in public places and immediately afterward, until you have a chance to wash your hands well. Surface transmission of the flu and other viruses is more common than transmission by sneezing or coughing. Many of the most concerning viruses can be transferred via public surfaces or people touching one another—such as shaking hands, touching door handles, using gas pumps, and sharing pens. If you use a public bathroom to wash up while you're out and about, use a paper towel to turn off the water and then to open the door to leave the bathroom, to keep your hands clean.

Keep preschool-age children at home. Childcare settings with large numbers of other children with runny noses are fertile ground for viruses, so don't use out-of-home childcare unless you have to. The last place you want to be with a sick child is an emergency room or a doctor's office, because these places will certainly increase your chances of getting an infectious disease.

If you do get the flu, stay home. Sip water all day, as opposed to guzzling a lot all at once. Eat as little as possible; if you're hungry, stick to light food, mostly juicy fruits and salads. Once you are ill, it is important not to overwork your body by making it digest heavy meals. Anorexia of infection (loss of appetite) is one way the body has of activating a more powerful immune response.

Knowing When to Call the Doctor

I do not recommend seeing a physician or seeking out medical assistance with typical flu or viral symptoms, such as a runny nose, fever, and body aches, because treating them with medications has no significant benefit. When a severe flu does occur, the main reason for hospitalization, severe illness, and even death is the complication of pneumonia. Instead of calling the doctor at the outset, watch for a sudden worsening of the overall condition, especially if worsening symptoms start to involve labored breathing. Symptoms suggesting that medical consultation is necessary are these:

- Rapid breathing

- Breathing with grunting or wheezing sounds

- Labored breathing (in a child, with rib muscles retracting)

- Abdominal pain (more common in children)

- Changes in behavior or mental status, such as disorientation or lack of alertness

- Persistent diarrhea or vomiting (more common with children), especially if unable to hold down sufficient fluids

- Persistent fever above 103 degrees for three days

Choose Nutrition over Medication

Remember that I mentioned the first pharmacology course I had in medical school, when the professor told us that all drugs are toxic? His words still ring true, and we physicians need to teach our patients how to avoid them. People do not build health via the ingestion of medicinal substances. Even natural, herbal products that have pharmacologic effects work because of their *toxic* properties, not their *nutritive* content. When you chose to live healthy, you limit your exposure to all treatments and remedies that could further compromise your long-term health.

It is important to understand that the choices you make today could punish you or protect you thirty to sixty years later. Health is complicated. All the contributory environmental factors leading to cancer are not yet known. However, we have learned much about cancer causation and the disease-fighting ability of a well-nourished immune system in recent years. We have the knowledge available today to do a much better job than our ancestors did at enhancing natural immunity, with a huge potential to extend our healthy life expectancy. I am of the opinion, based on my research and observation of patient outcomes over the last few decades, that most of us should be able to extend our lifespan to surpass ninety-five (good) years of age. However, we are not going to win the war on cancer or other life-threatening diseases with more medical treatments and more money devoted to medical care and drugs.

By adopting a protective lifestyle and diet, and making changes to improve our health and lower our risks of serious disease, we can reap substantial benefits. Only serious effort begets real and positive change, however. The same is true with anything in life. When we eat for Super Immunity, we protect ourselves not just from diseases, but also from the harmful effects of medications. Great health can be yours, but you can't buy it; you must earn it.

CHAPTER THREE

Super Foods
for Super Immunity

In May 2003, I was diagnosed with stage 4 non-Hodgkin's lymphoma. My physician at Sloan Kettering discussed with me the possible courses of action in treating my "chronic" and deadly disease. At that moment, one option was "wait and see," since I was not in immediate mortal danger. Somewhere up the road, it was suggested, I would probably need to take active measures, such as chemotherapy, to "manage" the disease. During the first panic-stricken days, my sister took me straight to Dr. Fuhrman. I believe the lessons I learned from the doctor over these past years have literally saved my life.

The first thing Dr. Fuhrman did was to explain to me how toxins that are linked to cancers such as mine are often lodged in people's fat tissues. He taught me how important it would be to lose weight and, with it, many of the toxins that might be causing cell dysfunction. In addition, he taught me what foods to avoid and what I needed to eat for optimal nutrition, what foods could help my body best to fight disease . . . and how to prepare them. When first I tasted a "blended salad," I lost my interest in eating altogether. But, now I

*love my high-nutrition meals. In addition to prescribing this
new way of eating, Dr. Fuhrman also recommended certain
supplements that would best complement my eating regimen.*

*I lost about forty pounds in the first three months of eat-
ing for life. My cholesterol level dropped from 238 to 164.
My other blood readings were excellent as well and have
remained so. And, in visit after visit to the oncologist, it did
not seem that my disease was advancing beyond the original tumor that was located in my groin. After two and a
half years of discussion about the possibility of undergoing
systemic chemotherapy, the tumor melted away, and has not
returned. In fact, no signs of the disease have been detected
since. And let's hope they won't be.*

*I don't think my energy levels were ever higher than they
are now, even as a youngster. And, at sixty-three years old,
I am a walking advertisement in support of Dr. Fuhrman's
brilliant approach to fighting disease and achieving optimal
health. I still report to my oncologist for periodic checkups,
and they are now pleasant enough. Tests regularly indicate that my body chemistry is normal and that there are
no tumors to be found. I consider myself a healthy woman
enjoying life to the max. And, although I wish no one harm,
I would not be surprised if I outlived the traditional oncolo-
gists I have met (unless of course they take the hint from me,
and begin attending to their nutrition!).*

—Irene Zabransky

Certain plant foods contain significant amounts of substances that
enhance human immune function and defenses against acute
illness and chronic disease. Creating delicious recipes and menus to
utilize these super foods is the eventual goal (see the final chapter);

however, learning why I include the foods I do, and why I mix and match certain foods together, is critical to your long-term success.

It has only been within the last ten years, more than thirty years after we landed the first man on the moon, that scientists have begun to identify certain compounds in plants that have powerful anticancer effects in humans.

More recently, the powerful anticancer and immune system–enhancing effects of greens, mushrooms, onions, pomegranates/berries, and seeds has been specifically noted by scientists. This new attention has led to testing in human studies. To date, in every study outcome, even a moderate amount of these foods offered significant benefits. For example, adding mushrooms to the diet lowers cancer rates, adding onions to the diet lowers cancer rates, adding greens to the diet lowers cancer rates, and adding blackberries to the diet lowers cancer rates.

However, my argument and recommendations are for people not just to eat these foods, but to eat these foods *in significant amounts and simultaneously*. The inevitable consequence of this shift to a diet with a range of immune system–strengthening and cancer-fighting foods is Super Immunity—immunity that can help you age in confidence, not fear, and in excellent health. We have to learn that illness and disease are not the inevitable consequences of aging, and that it is in our control *not* to get sick.

The line of research testing a combination of super foods in humans must continue, and certainly much more funding and support are needed. As we move forward with further studies and documented benefits of super foods, we don't want to miss the boat that is already pulling away from the dock right now, as a result of the preponderance of evidence available today. To stagnate in the muck, thinking that we don't have *sufficient* evidence yet, is a costly decision, and part of the reason why this book is so important.

My experience treating over ten thousand patients over the last twenty years using micronutrient-dense diets has demonstrated extraordinary therapeutic potential over a wide range of serious health conditions. I have seen the remarkable clinical response in a diverse patient population with diseases ranging from asthma and allergies, to heart disease and cancers, and have seen thousands of individuals improve and lengthen their lives. I strongly encourage you to start right now; don't wait until a health tragedy occurs that could have been averted.

The following case study reveals the incredible benefits of Super Immunity. I am *not* claiming that all or even most cases of advanced cancer can be reversed; however, I have had the fortunate experience to see dramatic cases like Pam's occur—cases demonstrating the power that superior nutrition has to enhance long-term survival.

CHILDREN'S BOOK AUTHOR PAMELA SWALLOW *sought my help in December 1997 when she learned that she had metastatic ovarian cancer that had spread into her lungs and abdomen. Her lungs had to be drained of fluid so she could breathe. Pam knew that she had to do everything possible to fight this normally deadly disease. The statistics for this type of cancer in stage 4 (which is where she was when I met her) show a five-year survival rate of only 10 percent and an even smaller ten-year survival rate.[1] This is because stage 4 ovarian cancer is difficult to completely remove with surgery, and the available chemotherapy is unable to eradicate all the remaining cancer.*

Pam had been told by several physicians that the only option for her in her difficult battle was chemotherapy and more surgery. Pam thought that nurturing and strengthening her immune system would be essential to her healing, so she investigated further; and soon she was referred to me.

After we spent time discussing all the ways the immune system has to fight cancer and attack isolated cancer cells as they recur, Pam began to feel more hopeful that she might live. Pam did go through chemotherapy for ovarian cancer, but when the treatments made her feel ill, she made green shakes, loaded with micronutrients. She and her husband began growing organic vegetables, and they bought an extra freezer so that they could keep for winter the produce that they weren't able to consume right away. What happened next is that Pam beat the statistics!

Today Pam still follows the immune-strengthening protocol I made for her fifteen years ago; she has not had any recurrence of cancer and has remained in excellent health. She says, "Dr. Fuhrman's approach to health is so sensible and rewarding, I can't imagine living any other way."

The Anticancer Solution

The process of "methylation" involves the addition of a simple four-atom molecule (one carbon and three hydrogen atoms, known as a "methyl group") to a gene.

Modification of human DNA by adding (or removing) these methyl groups on genes is associated with increased risk of cancer. In the science of cancer causation, it is well observed that methylation and demethylation create changes on the DNA molecule, and these changes occur early and ubiquitously in cancer development. When a gene is methylated or demethylated, it works differently than was intended—the methylation having turned either on or off certain parts of the DNA. As a result, methylation changes interfere with normal cell division, allowing some cells to grow wildly—which is cancer.

Consider the following interesting study conducted using over a thousand smokers or ex-smokers. They coughed up sputum from deep in their lungs to harvest lung tissue cells. The lung cells were analyzed for methylation in eight key genes, selected because those genes had been associated with cancer risk. Researchers counted cells with high methylation and used that as a marker for cancer risk. Then the researchers looked at the subjects' diets. They found that cancer risk, as defined by methylation in the cells, was lower in those who ate more leafy green vegetables.

It is very unusual to be born with DNA damage. That sort of damage builds up over time from exposure to toxins or a lack of micronutrients. The micronutrients in greens not only prevent such damage; they also repair and rebuild any damage that may have occurred.

The changes to a cell's DNA that lead to cancer are called "epigenetic." They are gradual changes that occur over time and accumulate until there is sufficient change to overcome normal cell control mechanisms. Cancer doesn't just pop up; it occurs after many years of self-abuse, and along this trail to carcinogenesis the changes can be stopped and repaired long before cells become cancerous.[2]

People who eat more leafy green vegetables have what we might call less risky DNA—less aberrant methylation—the studies find. The methylation phenomenon, its link with cancer, and the prevention of aberrant methylation by green vegetables has been noted in various studies as well.[3] The phytochemical compounds in green vegetables—remember our earlier discussion?—not only prevent aberrant methylation and demethylation but actually enable cell repair mechanisms to repair improperly methylated segments of the DNA.

Here's how the proposed model works:

More Green Vegetables ⟶ Less DNA Methylation ⟶ Lower Risk of Cancer

This can also be expressed in an opposite model:

Less Green Vegetables ⟶ More DNA Methylation ⟶ Higher Risk of Cancer

Cruciferous Disease Fighters

Green vegetables such as kale, cabbage, collards, and broccoli, plus some nongreen vegetables such as cauliflower and turnips, are called "cruciferous" vegetables. They are named for their flowers, which have four equally spaced petals in the shape of a cross—hence the Latin word *crucifer,* meaning "cross-bearer." *All* vegetables contain protective micronutrients and phytochemicals, but cruciferous vegetables have a unique chemical composition: they have sulfur-containing compounds that are responsible for their pungent or bitter flavors. When their cell walls are broken by blending or chopping, a chemical reaction occurs that converts these sulfur-containing compounds into isothiocyanates (ITCs)—an array of compounds with proven and powerful immune-boosting effects and anticancer activity.

Cruciferous Vegetables as Anticancer Agents

Over 120 ITCs have been identified, and the various ITCs have different mechanisms of action. Because different ITCs work in different locations in the cell, and on different molecules, they can have combined additive effects, working synergistically to remove carcinogens and kill cancer cells. Furthermore, some ITCs have anti-inflammatory, antioxidant, or even immunologic effects. ITCs can inhibit angiogenesis, the process by which a tumor promotes blood vessel growth to feed its multiplying and growing cancer cells with nourishment. Cancer-prone and malignant cells secrete factors that stimulate new blood vessel growth, thus promoting their own survival and spread. A fundamental step in the transition to cancer is the successful promotion of blood vessels, so foods that inhibit angiogenesis are well-recognized and powerful cancer fighters. (We'll talk more about this when we get to mushrooms!)

Certain ITCs detoxify and/or remove carcinogenic compounds—especially the green cruciferous vegetables, such as broccoli and brussels sprouts, which are rich sources of the ITC sulforaphane.[4] Sulforaphane prevents carcinogens from binding to the DNA and being able to initiate cancerous changes in the cell, and it activates enzymes that protect cells from any DNA damage that has occurred.[5] ITCs give each cell its own protective shield, isolating destructive toxins and neutralizing or compartmentalizing them so that they cannot do damage. But if DNA does indeed become damaged, the growth of a damaged cell can be stopped to allow for DNA repair, or the cell can be programmed for cell death (again, "apoptosis").

The processes that protect the inside of cells from damage can only be fueled by these compounds in green vegetables. Several ITCs, including sulforaphane, indole-3-carbinol, and diindolylmethane, have been studied for their purported ability to stop growth or induce death in cancer cells such as those involved in breast and colon cancer.[6] Other ITCs with strong anticancer activity include phenylethyl-isothiocyanate (PEITC) and allyl isothiocyanate (AITC).

Apparently, the human body is already programmed to fight infection and fight off cancer. The immune system is like a protective force field in a sci-fi movie, but hardly anybody turns it on because they don't fuel the force-field engine, which runs on greens.

Indole-3-carbinol (I3C) and its metabolite diindolylmethane (DIM) may be especially protective against hormone-sensitive cancers; they help the body transform estrogen and other hormones into forms that are more easily excreted from the body.[7] Metabolites such as DIM are formed as part of the natural biochemical process of degrading and eliminating their parent compound.

These observations in cell culture and animal studies have been confirmed by human epidemiological studies that look at the connections between cruciferous vegetable intake and cancer incidence. As cruciferous vegetable intake increases, breast, lung, prostate, and colorectal cancers decrease accordingly. Similar associations linking total vegetable intake to lower cancer incidence have been noted, but cruciferous vegetables are far more potent and have a more profound association in the scientific literature. Note the following specifics:

- Cruciferous vegetables are twice as powerful as other plant foods. In population studies, a 20 percent increase in plant food intake generally corresponds to a 20 percent decrease in cancer rates, but a 20 percent increase in *cruciferous* vegetable intake corresponds to a 40 percent decrease in cancer rates.[8]

- Twenty-eight servings of vegetables per week decreases prostate cancer risk by 33 percent, but just three servings of *cruciferous* vegetables per week decreases prostate cancer risk by 41 percent.[9]

- One or more servings of cabbage per week reduces the occurrence of pancreatic cancer by 38 percent.[10]

Cruciferous Vegetables as Antiviral and Antibacterial Agents

Now here's where this gets even more interesting. Not only do I3C and DIM offer dramatic protective effects against cancer, but recent studies have shown that these ITCs are important in enabling interferon responsiveness, which serves as a potent immune-system stimulator to attack microbes such as viruses. Specifically, these ITCs have been shown to increase the immune system's cell-killing capacity and heighten resistance to viral infection, with impressive results.[11] DIM has already been shown to resolve cervical dysplasia, laryngeal papillomas, and warts. It is presently under investigational study as a treatment for a variety of viral infections and antibiotic-resistant bacteria, including HIV (human immunodeficiency virus), HPV (human papilloma virus), and hepatitis.[12]

Of critical interest here is also that cruciferous-derived compounds work together to enhance defenses against bacterial infections, especially with the ability of certain bacteria to develop resistance to antibiotics. Of particular concern are hospital-contracted (i.e., "nosocomial") infections, which exhibit antibiotic resistance. The bacterium known as *Streptococcus pneumoniae,* for example, causes approximately 3,000 cases of meningitis, 50,000 cases of bacteremia, 500,000 cases of pneumonia, and nearly 7,000,000 cases of otitis media in the United States, in addition to being a leading cause of mortality. Antibiotic-resistant strains of streptococcus have emerged and are now becoming widespread in certain communities. ITC compounds from greens have natural antimicrobial effects that can be utilized as an aid to boost natural cellular defenses, enabling a heightened state of resistance against these dangerous drug-resistant bacteria.[13]

These same green-vegetable-derived compounds also fight against *Helicobacter pylori.* This bacterium is a contributory factor to ulcer disease and is associated with a marked increase in the risk of stomach cancer. A high consumption of cruciferous greens inhibits *H. pylori:* when their ITC compounds have been tested, they have shown potential as a novel treatment for conditions caused by this bacterium.[14] Even though this research has been conducted mostly in animals, with only a limited number of human participants, it contributes to the point here: the regular consumption of all these micronutrients in greens builds up a *constellation* of beneficial health effects that reduce one's chance of contracting infections and increase one's chance of overcoming them.

Another example of the protective power of cruciferous greens occurs with Nrf2, a master regulator of the antioxidant response. This complex protein, a so-called transcription factor, activates our genes to produce a broad array of protective compounds that shield against inflammation and disease.

How does this happen? Waste products in cells age us prematurely and create disease, as we saw in the earlier discussion of free radicals. There are two types of waste: *exogenous* waste that we ingest from the external environment and *endogenous* waste that builds up as a by-product of cellular metabolism. The presence and function of the Nrf2 transcription factor is critical for endogenous detoxification and free-radical scavenging. Endogenous wastes, also referred to as "reactive oxygen species" (ROS), can damage biological macromolecules and thus are detrimental to cellular health. They are called "reactive" because of their free radicals, which multiply in human tissue and cause destruction of normal cellular structures. If not rapidly removed, these reactive compounds cause disease and premature aging. It's as if a tornado were growing in strength inside your home, eventually tearing it apart from the inside out.

We are protected against these reactive wastes by a series of proteins coded for by genes that contain sequences called "antioxidant response elements" (ARE). The Nrf2 proteins are transcription factors that bind to and activate the ARE segments of genes. These genes activate the body's own protective response, which then protects us from a variety of oxidative stress–related complications, even in situations where the administration of exogenous antioxidants, which are short-acting (such as vitamin C and vitamin E), fail. Nrf2 becomes activated (a normal function) when we eat green vegetables supplying ITCs. When we don't eat cruciferous greens, one of the most important natural defense systems in the cell (Nrf2–ARE) simply does not function. More evidence that we are dependent on the substances in greens for longevity and excellent health!

The Nrf2 factor is also responsible for preventing deposits of plaque in the inside of blood vessels. The endothelial cells that line the blood vessels are able to prevent adhesion by inflammatory cells that promote plaque formation when Nrf2 is activated. That's why green vegetables are so important for heart health (and even to promote reversal of heart disease): they activate the Nrf2 factor. Nrf2 then changes the proteins expressed on the endothelial cell membranes, preventing atherosclerosis deposits from forming there. Activating Nrf2 is especially critical to coronary vessels at bifurcation or curves with increased pressure, where plaque is more likely to build.[15]

Maximizing the Benefits of Cruciferous Vegetables

Methods of preparation and cooking affect the availability of ITCs to be digested and absorbed. Chopping, chewing, blending, and juicing all allow for enhanced production of ITCs. In other words, these beneficial ITCs are not preformed in the plant; they are made in our mouth from glucosinolate precursors as we chew and crush the cell walls. The more cell walls that are broken, the more myrosinase (an enzyme housed in the cell membrane) that is released and can be mixed with the glucosinolates inside the cell to catalyze the reaction that makes ITCs.

Some ITC benefit may be lost with boiling or steaming, as the myrosinase enzyme can be destroyed with too much heat; so we get

INOLATES + MYROSINASE = ISOTHIOCYANATES (ITCS)

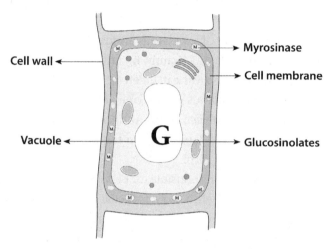

Cell wall — Myrosinase

Cell membrane

Vacuole — G — Glucosinolates

the maximum benefit from eating cruciferous vegetables raw. However, some production of ITC in cooked cruciferous vegetables may still occur, because the bacteria in the digestive tract have some myrosinase activity. The myrosinase-producing ability of gut bacteria can be increased with the regular consumption of—you guessed it!—green vegetables.

Keep in mind that cooking does not destroy the activity and function of the ITCs; it only deactivates the enzyme catalyzing their formation. That means if you blend, crush, chop, or juice the greens while they're raw to maximize the ITC production and then put the blended or chopped greens into a stew or soup to cook, you will still have those functioning and beneficial ITCs present after cooking.

To maximize the immune-function benefits of cruciferous vegetables, do the following:

1. Chew all cruciferous greens very, very well, trying to crush every cell.

2. Puree, blend, or chop cruciferous vegetables before adding them to stews or soups.

3. When steaming green cruciferous vegetables such as broccoli and cabbage, try to undercook slightly so they are not too mushy.

Cruciferous vegetables are not only the most powerful anticancer foods in existence; they are also the most micronutrient-dense of all vegetables. Although the National Cancer Institute recommends five to nine servings of fruits and vegetables per day for cancer prevention, they have not yet established specific recommendations for cruciferous vegetables. I recommend three fresh fruits and eight total servings of vegetables per day, including two servings of cruciferous vegetables (at least one raw). Consuming a large variety of these ITC-rich cruciferous vegetables within an overall nutrient-dense diet can provide a profound level of protection against infection and cancer.

CRUCIFEROUS VEGETABLES

Arugula	Cabbage	Mustard greens
Bok choy	Cauliflower	Radishes
Broccoli	Collards	Red cabbage
Broccoli rabe	Horseradish	Turnip greens
Broccolini	Kale	Watercress
Brussels sprouts	Kohlrabi	

Life-Saving Mushrooms

Among the amazing super foods that play an important role in keeping the immune system strong are mushrooms. Mushrooms are unique: they contain many unusual disease-fighting compounds that are just beginning to be understood.

There are several immune-supporting ingredients in mushrooms that empower the body to react quickly and powerfully when we are exposed to disease-causing pathogens such as viruses and bacteria. In most cases, we can defeat the microbes we are exposed to before any symptoms occur. Mushroom phytochemicals may even be helpful for autoimmune diseases such as rheumatoid arthritis and lupus because of their anti-inflammatory and immune-modulating effects.[16]

If green vegetables are the king of Super Immunity, mushrooms are the queen. First of all, the compounds found in simple mushrooms have been shown in animal experiments and cell cultures to enhance the activity and function of natural killer T cells (NKT).[17] NKTs detect cells infected with a virus or damaged in some way, and attack and remove them. Activated NKT cells attack the abnormal cells by releasing "killing granules" to destroy abnormal cells.

White, cremini, portobello, oyster, maitake, and reishi mushrooms have all been shown to have anticancer effects: they prevent DNA damage, slow cancer cell or tumor growth, cause programmed cancer cell death, and/or prevent tumors from acquiring a blood supply. These effects have been shown in breast, prostate, and colon cancers and/or cancer cells.[18]

Common mushrooms contain antigen-binding lectins (ABL), proteins that bind only to abnormal cells by recognizing a molecule on the surface of many cancer cells and then activating the body's defenses, calling them into action against those cells.[19] Interestingly, after these lectins are attracted to and bind to an abnormal cell, they then become internalized into the cell and interfere with the cell's ability to replicate itself, thus preventing the spread of cancer, without having any toxicity or negative effects on normal cells.

Winning the War on Breast Cancer

Consuming mushrooms regularly is associated with a significantly decreased risk of breast cancer in both pre- and postmenopausal women. Amazingly, frequent consumption of mushrooms can decrease the incidence of breast cancer by up to 60 to 70 percent! In one recent study, women who ate at least 10 grams of fresh mushrooms each day (equivalent to just one small mushroom) had a 64 percent decreased risk of breast cancer. Even more dramatic protection was gained by women who ate 10 grams of mushrooms and consumed green compounds from green tea daily—an 89 percent decrease in risk for premenopausal women and 82 percent for postmenopausal women.[20] Similar associations were observed in studies on stomach and colorectal cancers.[21] Hard to believe, isn't it? Why doesn't *every* woman know the protective effects that mushrooms have against breast cancer? The combination of mushrooms and greens is a powerful anticancer cocktail.

Mushrooms fight breast cancer in many ways. They contain compounds called "aromatase inhibitors" that help the body reduce the level of estrogen and prevent estrogen from stimulating breast tissue.[22] Aromatase (sometimes called "estrogen synthase") is an enzyme that produces estrogen and is responsible for regulating estrogen levels in the body. Since estrogen plays an important role in the development of breast cancer, suppression of aromatase activity is protective. Excessive expression of the aromatase enzyme in breast tumors is thought to contribute to the progression of breast cancers by elevating estrogen levels in the surrounding area.[23]

There are currently drugs used as therapies for certain cancers that inhibit aromatase activity.[24] But dietary aromatase inhibitors are an effective lifetime preventive strategy that will dampen estrogen levels, reducing breast cancer risk. Several varieties of mushrooms have been tested for their anti-aromatase activity. This is how they ranked:

- High anti-aromatase activity: white button, white stuffing, cremini, portobello, reishi, maitake
- Mild anti-aromatase activity: shiitake, chanterelle, baby button
- Little or no anti-aromatase activity: oyster, wood ear[25]

Regardless of anti-aromatase activity, the beneficial anti–breast cancer action in mushrooms was found in all species of mushrooms tested and was heat-stable, meaning that it continued to be effective even after the mushrooms were cooked. The most common and least expensive mushrooms—white button mushrooms—showed these strong benefits. If that's not enough great news about mushrooms, there's more.

Mushrooms as Team Players

Mushrooms promote the body's production and maturation of dendritic cells and improve their antigen-presenting function.[26] Let's take that apart. Dendritic cells are tree-shaped immune cells that are scattered throughout the body in their immature or deactivated form. When activated, they trap and process what they recognize as enemy material, presenting it to other immune cells to remove or kill the threat. In other words, they capture microbial pathogens and abnormal cells so that other immune cells can destroy them.

Dendritic cells are present in tissues in contact with the external environment, such as the skin and the inner lining of the nose, lungs, stomach, and intestines. They can also be found in an immature state in the blood. Once activated and engaged, they migrate to the lymph nodes, where they interact with T cells and B cells to initiate an immune attack.

Dendritic cell functions can decrease with aging, leading to a loss of immune function. This gradual loss in dendritic function exposes us to infection and a higher risk of developing cancer as we get older. However, the ingestion of the immune-strengthening compounds derived from mushrooms and greens can prevent this age-related loss of immune function.[27]

Even though mushrooms have unique phytochemical compounds with a host of unique immune-strengthening effects, their ability is further enhanced when the diet contains mushrooms, onions, and green vegetables simultaneously. Not only mushrooms, but phytochemicals called "flavonoids," found in colorful fruits, onions, and berries, as well the green-vegetable-derived isothiocyanates (ITCs), have been identified as anticarcinogens, capable of activating dendritic cells.[28]

Mushrooms also contain an angiogenesis inhibitor that further inhibits tumors and growth of abnormal cells, tumors, and cancers.

Angiogenesis, as you may recall, means the growth of new blood vessels. Cancers, tumors, and fat secrete angiogenesis-promoting compounds that fuel their own growth; but mushrooms say no.

ANGIOGENESIS—A NECESSARY STEP IN FEEDING THE GROWTH OF BODY FAT AND CANCER

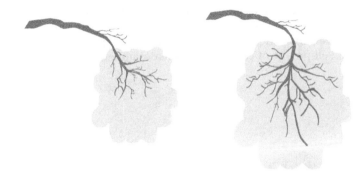

Angiogenesis is a complex physiological process by which new blood vessels are formed from previously existing ones. In response to an angiogenic signal, endothelial cells sprout from the original blood vessel, divide, and form tubelike structures that mature into new vessels. Angiogenesis occurs during fetal development and normal childhood growth. In adults, angiogenesis occurs only in certain specific situations, like wound healing. However, excessive (i.e., abnormal) angiogenesis contributes to several disease states, such as obesity, cancer, macular degeneration, and chronic inflammatory conditions.

In cancer development, angiogenesis is initiated when a tumor becomes large enough to need its own blood supply. The tumor signals nearby blood vessels to branch off and supply it with oxygen and nutrients, and these new vessels allow a nonthreatening microscopic tumor to grow and become invasive and dangerous. The hallmark of cancer is the rapid, uncontrolled growth and replication of cells; that is what makes cancer life-threatening. Since angiogenesis is rare in healthy adults and necessary for tumor growth, blocking angiogenesis is a strategy in cancer prevention and treatment. Several drugs have been developed that were designed to block different steps of the angiogenic process, and some of these drugs have been approved by the FDA and are currently being used as cancer therapies.[29]

ANGIOGENESIS INHIBITION	ANGIOGENESIS PROMOTION
Prevents tumors from growing	Promotes tumors and cancers
Prevents fat cells from expanding	Promotes fat deposition
Prevents inflammation	Increases inflammation
Inhibits development of cancer	Increases appetite

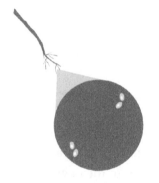 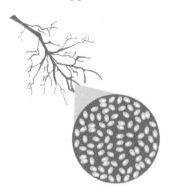

Many plant foods contain natural angiogenesis inhibitors—especially mushrooms. Dietary angiogenesis inhibitors are now being investigated as a preventive strategy to "starve" cancers while they are still small and harmless. If our diet contains plenty of angiogenesis inhibitors, it can prevent small tumors from acquiring a blood supply and growing larger and becoming more aggressive or cancerous. This is one more way that mushrooms, onions, greens, and berries—preferably in conjunction—protect against cancer.

As a safety precaution, mushrooms should always be consumed cooked, since some studies have reported toxic effects of raw mushrooms in animal studies.[30]

ANTI-ANGIOGENIC FOODS/NUTRIENTS

Allium vegetables (onion family)[32]	Omega-3 fats[43]
Berries (all types)[33]	Peppers[44]
Black rice[34]	Pomegranate[45]
Cinnamon[35]	Quince[46]
Citrus fruits[36]	Resveratrol (from grapes and
Cruciferous vegetables[37]	red wine)
Flax seeds[38]	Soybeans[47]
Ginger[39]	Spinach[48]
Grapes[40]	Tomatoes[49]
Green tea[41]	Turmeric[50]
Mushrooms[42]	

These foods are listed in alphabetical order, not in the order of their angiogenesis-inhibiting effects.

Stopping the Growth of Fat Cells

Similarly, the growth of fat tissue is dependent on angiogenesis, and inhibition of angiogenesis through the consumption of beneficial angiogenesis-inhibiting foods inhibits fat deposition and growth.[31] That means eating these super foods, with mushrooms leading the way, has the side effect of encouraging a healthy weight. That occurs not just because of the lower calorie density of such a diet, but also because of other beneficial nutrients ingested, including angiogenesis inhibitors.

Foods and nutrients that *promote* angiogenesis—and thus obesity and cancer—include white-flour based breads and sweets that raise insulin levels, and the high-fat, high-cholesterol, standard Western diet.[51] These modern, unhealthy foods promote fat storage in addition to having a high-caloric density. They are a double negative, while greens, mushrooms, onions, berries, and the other foods listed above are a double positive.

Onions and Garlic:
Anticancer and Immunity-Building Treasures

The allium family of vegetables, which includes onions, garlic, leeks, shallots, chives, and scallions, adds more than just flavor to your diet; its members also add anticancer, anti-inflammatory, and antioxidant compounds. Even far back in history, people were well aware that these foods had medicinal value and consumed them on a daily basis. In medieval times, for example, people recognized that onions and garlic offered immune protection and would help them get well faster in the event that they did come down with an infection. We have lost touch with using food as medicine, but the right natural foods are truly our most effective remedies.

Epidemiological studies have found that increased consumption of allium vegetables is associated with lower risk of cancer at all common sites. This protection is thought to be due to their organosulfur compounds, which are released when the vegetables are chopped, crushed, or chewed. Similar to the green cruciferous family, the cell walls of onions house an enzyme called alliinase, which is responsible for making that sulfuric acid smell that can make you cry. At the same time the chemical reaction is occurring on your kitchen counter and smarting your eyes, those immune-building sulfide compounds are forming. These compounds prevent the development of cancers by detoxifying carcinogens, and they also have angiogenesis-inhibiting effects that halt cancer cell growth by preventing tumors from obtaining a blood supply.[52]

New research suggests that these organosulfur compounds in members of the onion family also have anti-inflammatory actions that protect against osteoarthritis and ward off infections. When we eat the organosulfur compounds and glycoproteins in onions, those compounds work together with other micronutrients to improve immune function and to prevent disease. In fact, when onion intake was scrutinized in a case-control multicountry study, the highest consumers of onions had less than half as many cancers compared to people who rarely consumed onions. Here are the specific stats:[53]

- A 56 percent reduction in colon cancer
- A 73 percent reduction in ovarian cancer
- An 88 percent reduction in esophageal cancer
- A 71 percent reduction in prostate cancer
- A 50 percent reduction in stomach cancer

In this study the highest consumers were eating seven or more 80 gram portions per week (or about ½ cup of chopped onions per day); the lowest consumers were eating less than one serving per week. Imagine the protective effects of eating adequate amounts of the top three super food groups *together*—cruciferous greens, mushrooms, and onions—almost daily.

Pomegranates and Berries: Superheroes in Disguise

The pomegranate is a unique ancient fruit borne on a small, long-living tree cultivated throughout Asia and the Mediterranean region, as far north as the Himalayas. As a result of the increasing recognition of its health benefits, it is now also grown in California and elsewhere in the southern United States.

In the past decade, numerous studies on the antioxidant, anticarcinogenic, and anti-inflammatory properties of pomegranates have been published, focusing on the treatment and prevention of cancer, cardiovascular disease, diabetes, erectile dysfunction, bacterial infections and antibiotic resistance, and ultraviolet radiation–induced skin damage.[54]

The juice and seeds of the pomegranate possess potent antioxidant and anticancer properties, including interference with tumor cell proliferation, cell cycle–dependent invasion, and angiogenesis. The phytochemistry of pomegranates suggests a wide range of clinical applications for the treatment and prevention of cancer, as well as other diseases in which chronic inflammation is believed to play an essential role. Pomegranate juice contains antioxidants such as soluble polyphenols, tannins, and anthocyanins, and has been shown to have anti-inflammatory, antibacterial, and anti-atherosclerotic properties in mice and humans.

The following list highlights some of the benefits of pomegranate seeds and juice, as revealed by recent research:

1. Pomegranates inhibit breast cancer, prostate cancer, colon cancer, and leukemia, and prevent vascular changes that promote tumor growth in lab animals.[55]

2. Pomegranates inhibit angiotensin-converting enzymes and naturally lower blood pressure. (Angiotensin, as you may recall, is a hormone that promotes angiogenesis.)[56]

HOW TO OPEN A POMEGRANATE

Purchase a firm fruit. Keep it refrigerated until use, for freshness. Cut around the center (the "equator," if you will), inserting the knife about half an inch all the way around; then twist the fruit apart, separating it into two halves.

Hold the half pomegranate in your cupped hand, with the cut side down, and position that hand over a large salad bowl. Using the side of a heavy wooden spoon, bang the pomegranate hard all around the top dome, around the middle, and all around the bottom edge close to your hand. Give every square inch a good hit. You should be able to see the skin softening and bending as you smack it, and feel the small red seeds falling past your hand and into the salad bowl. Now take the softened skin and invert it—turn it inside out—to remove any remaining seeds with your fingers. Repeat for the other side.

Eat your pomegranate seeds plain, use them in salads and recipes, or freeze them for later use, when they are out of season. There are some great ideas in the recipes at the end of the book to help you enjoy pomegranates *often* in your eating plan.

3. The potent antioxidative compounds in pomegranates reverse atherosclerosis and reduce excessive blood clotting and platelet clumping, factors that can lead to heart attacks and strokes.[57]

4. Pomegranates have estrogen-like compounds that stimulate serotonin and estrogen receptors, improving symptoms of depression and helping build bone mass in lab animals.[58]

5. Pomegranates reduce tissue damage in those with kidney problems, reduce the incidence of infections, and prevent serious infections.[59]

6. Lastly but impressively, pomegranates improve heart health. Heart patients with severe carotid artery blockages were given a daily dose of less than an ounce of pomegranate juice for a year. Not only did their blood pressure decrease by over 20 percent, but there was a 30 percent reduction in atherosclerotic plaque.[60]

Interestingly, pomegranates offer significant active protection against breast cancer. Like mushrooms, they support anti-aromatase activity; that means they prevent estrogen and testosterone from rising too high in the body and block the stimulation of breast tissues with these hormones.[61] An increasing body of evidence has underscored the cancer-preventive efficacy of pomegranates in animal models and human studies.[62]

Colorful berries have beneficial effects similar to those of pomegranates. Consider the following research: after exposure to a chemical carcinogen that damages DNA in rats, the animals were fed dried blackberries and showed a transformation of the damaged genes back to near-normal; the effects were just as marked as the benefits from cruciferous greens.[63] The model of exposing rats to chemical carcinogens and then giving them berries has been repeated in many other studies as well, and exposure to berries or berry concentrates repeatedly shows a reduction in the occurrence of cancer at multiple sites, including esophagus, colon, and oral cancers. Similarly, when rats were implanted with estrogen to produce mammary tumors, blueberry and raspberry intake was able to limit the development of the tumors to begin with, and once tumors were induced, the berry extracts reduced tumor size.

The idea of berries as anticarcinogens was first conceived in the late 1980s, when scientists discovered that ellagic acid, found in many fruits and vegetables (including pomegranates), inhibited the formations of tumors. They then found that berries contained *markedly* high amounts of ellagic acid, and that black raspberries in particular had the most among berries and fruits. Later it was found that berries also contained many other anticancer phytochemical compounds, such as an assortment of anthocyanins with powerful anticancer effects.[64] All berries and their juices—including blueberries, blackberries, raspberries, acai berries, goji berries, elderberries, and strawberries—are super foods.

Seeds: A New Door to Great Health

Before we close this chapter on super foods, I must discuss the value of nuts and seeds, which we looked at briefly in a previous chapter. They are high in fat and protein, like animal products, but their effects on the body are completely different. Instead of promoting disease, as animal protein and animal fat do, they actually prevent and reverse it. They have been demonstrated in hundreds of medical studies to dramatically extend life and protect against disease.[65]

Nuts and seeds are not only tasty and healthy foods; they are portable and easy to take along while traveling. How else could you carry half a day's calories in your computer case on a business trip or in your daypack while on an all-day hike?

Seeds give you all the advantages of nuts, plus more. They are higher in protein than nuts and have many additional important nutrients, making them a particularly wonderful food. Unlike Wonder Bread, they really do build strong bodies twelve ways. Each seed is a living but rugged food, sealed in a package that, amazingly, can still germinate after two hundred years if stored in favorable conditions! Let's look at what various kinds of seeds have to offer:

Flax seeds don't just give you omega-3 fatty acids (essential for good health); they are also rich in anticancer lignans, and their mucilage lubricates and eases bowel movements. Flax seeds and sesame seeds contain more lignans than any other food. These plant compounds bind to estrogen receptors and interfere with the cancer-promoting effects of estrogen on breast tissue and they also have strong antioxidant effects. You can purchase flax seeds already ground and ready to eat, however it is best to grind your own fresh at home. Of special interest is a study that revealed that when flax seeds are given to women with breast cancer, the women show reduced tumor growth and enhanced survival, compared to women not given flax.[66]

Sunflower seeds are exceedingly rich in vitamin E, selenium, iron, and other minerals. With 22 percent of calories from protein and rich in the amino acid tryptophan, sunflower seeds are a healthy way that vegetarians, vegans, flexitarians (near-vegans), and nutritarians can ensure that they get sufficient protein.

Pumpkin seeds are a good source of omega-3s, are high in phyto-chemicals, and are rich in zinc, calcium, and iron.

Sesame seeds have the highest level of calcium of any food in the world. Interestingly, they not only have a highly absorbable full spectrum of various vitamin E fractions, but they increase the bioactivity of vitamin E in the body.[67]

Natural vitamin E is a complex, fat-soluble chemical structure that includes alpha-, beta-, gamma-, and delta-tocopherols and tocotrienols, present in the leaves and seeds of plants. It is not only a potent antioxidant and free-radical scavenger, but it also

Top Super Foods for Super Immunity

Kale/collards/mustard greens	Mushrooms
Arugula/watercress	Pomegranates
Green lettuce and cabbage	Berries (all types)
Broccoli and brussels sprouts,	Seeds (flax, chia, sesame,
Carrots and tomatoes	sunflower)
Onions and garlic	

regulates immune system activity and is essential for life. Its benefits are not equaled by synthetic vitamin E supplements, which typically include only one or two vitamin E isomers. Comparing the many forms of vitamin E in sesame seeds to the vitamin E in a supplement is like comparing a real horse to a toy horse. Sesamin, a sesame lignan, also has beneficial effects to improve postmenopausal hormonal status, raise antioxidant activity in body cells, and at the same time decrease the risk of breast cancer and lower cholesterol.[68]

The Micronutrient Revolution

We have an opportunity to earn great health via what we eat. The powerful compounds found in nuts and seeds, berries, and pomegranates are potently protective; when they are combined with green vegetables, mushrooms, and onions in the diet, that aggregate begets Super Immunity, fueling the miraculous self-healing and self-protective properties already built into the human genome. A combination of these compounds is far more effective than any single agent, even in a high dose. Acting together, they fuel an assortment of mechanisms that both prevent cell damage and also kill cells that cannot be adequately repaired before they can become dangerous to the body.

This nutritarian approach, which mixes the most powerful and protective foods in the diet, is natural, is without toxicity, and can prevent many human tragedies—not just revving up our immune system against infection and cancer, but also preventing heart attacks, strokes, and dementia. The line of research testing a combination of super foods in humans needs much more funding and support. If it received that support, we would certainly find that a whole range of high-micronutrient super foods have a wide range of therapeutic possibilities against serious health conditions.

In the case of every one of the super foods, a moderate amount alone offers substantial benefits. However, as noted earlier, my argument and recommendations are for people to eat significant protective amounts of these super foods, and to include them *all* (or most of them) in your diet. Super Immunity is created by a diet with a portfolio of immune system–strengthening and cancer-fighting foods. Here's a good way to remember the essentials:

GBOMBS
Greens, beans, onions, mushrooms, berries, seeds
Greens, beans, onions, mushrooms, berries, seeds
Greens, beans, onions, mushrooms, berries, seeds

Nutritional science has provided us an unprecedented opportunity. We can live healthier and longer than at any point in human history if we put this science into action. We are living in an age of scientific advancements of all kinds. But science is a double-edged sword; it can cure us or destroy us. It can answer our questions, or create more problems. My hope is that we can learn to use modern advancements in science to benefit humanity and protect our natural environment from chemical and physical destruction. Clearly, our health is dependent on the health of our planet and on sustaining a healthy supply of natural, unadulterated food.

Many people choose to reject new science, even when the evidence is overwhelming. This book may be attacked by people in powerful positions of authority whose livelihood is dependent on competing interests, such as "recreational" foods, drugs, and medical technology. Too often people mistake authority for truth: they accept an opinion voiced by a person of high authority, right or wrong, instead of undertaking an unbiased scrutiny of the facts. Doctors are guilty of this all the time. They accept conclusions fed to them by prestigious medical journals about studies that were performed by drug companies promoting their products, without an adequate awareness of the bias in the study preparation. In order to help ourselves, our families, our neighbors, our nation, and our fellow earthlings, we have to cultivate a respect for the precious value of our natural world while also cultivating the best natural foods that can protect our precious health.

CHAPTER FOUR

Colds and Flu—
What We Need to Know

The common cold continues to be a great burden on society, in terms of both human suffering and economic loss.

The common cold, the flu, and over 95 percent of all acute sicknesses are caused by viruses. I mention this specifically because one of the major issues with colds and flu is not the illness itself but the myriad ways we try to treat it. Too often these so-called solutions tax our immune system, prolonging the illness, or turning colds and flu into something much worse, even potentially life-threatening.

Everyone should be aware by now that antibiotics do *not* kill viruses and do *not* aid in the recovery from viral illness. Yet over 90 percent of antibiotic prescriptions are utilized inappropriately (that is, prescribed for viral illnesses). That's right, 90 percent! Antibiotics are routinely and repeatedly administered by physicians for illnesses such as colds and bronchitis, which are viral, not bacterial.[1] In one study, more than half of the patients who visited a physician in the United States with cold symptoms left with a prescription for an antibiotic.[2] This use of antibiotics is inappropriate and dangerous.

The common cold is caused by a host of viral invaders. The primary offenders are the so-called rhinoviruses, but others include coronavirus, parainfluenza virus, respiratory syncytial virus, adenovirus, echovirus, and coxsackievirus. Typically, the common cold is contracted by touching a contaminated object or shaking the hand of an infected person, and then touching one's eyes, nose, or mouth.

Influenza, on the other hand, is caused by one of three types of influenza virus: A, B, or C. It is contracted primarily through inhalation, when an uninfected person is close to an infected person who is sneezing or coughing.

The vast majority of sore throats (pharyngitis), sinus congestion and drainage (sinusitis), and bad coughs (bronchitis) are of viral causation. It is well established that antibiotics are not helpful in these conditions; they are useful only in relatively rare cases, such as bronchitis in smokers, or in former smokers with lung disease who are prone to developing bacterial overgrowth when infected.[3] The misuse of antibiotics is a multibillion-dollar industry in the United States every year.

A common misconception exists among those suffering from cold and/or flu symptoms regarding the color of the mucous: many people believe that yellow- or green-tinted mucous indicates bacterial involvement (thus calling for antibiotic treatment). This is an important point: research has shown that patients do *not* benefit from antibiotics even in the presence of green or thick sputum.[4] That is, the color of the sputum was not found to be an indicator of bacterial involvement; viral pathogens also produce thick yellow- or green-tinted mucous.

So when you have a cold, a fever, a sore throat, body aches, and nasal congestion, and are coughing up thick yellow or green mucous, medications are *not* indicated and are *not* supported by the scientific data. In fact, medication will not help you get better faster and will not prevent further complications.

Besides their ineffectiveness, there are other compelling reasons to avoid the use of antibiotics. They can actually prolong your illness—but worse, they can lead to more serious illnesses in your future. The problem is that when we get sick, when we become physically very uncomfortable, we look for a solution. That's human nature: no one wants to feel miserable, and we all have things that must get done in our busy lives. So we look to over-the-counter medications; or even worse, we go to a physician seeking more powerful drugs for relief.

Unfortunately, most physicians seem to comply, wanting to meet their patients' expectations. They assume the role of "savior," when in fact their antibiotic prescriptions not only are not helpful, but more likely are harmful to patients' long-term health. Increased hospitalizations attributed to adverse drug reactions alone account for billions of dollars each year within the U.S. health care system. Over 140,000 of these severe reactions to antibiotics drive people to emergency rooms each year; and they are not just costly financially, but serious and even tragic in human terms.[5] Antibacterial adverse effects account for nearly 25 percent of all adverse drug reactions among hospitalized patients.[6]

If that doesn't make you think twice about the inappropriate use of antibiotics, consider that antibiotics can cause cancer. A history of using antibiotics more than ten times in childhood increases the likelihood of developing non-Hodgkin's lymphoma (NHL) by 80 percent, according to the largest case-controlled study to date of NHL risk and medication use.[7] Other studies looking at this issue also confirm a link to cancer, including a higher rate of breast cancer, which increased as prescriptions for antibiotics increased.[8] The investigators found that increasing the cumulative days of antibiotic use and the cumulative number of antibiotic prescriptions increased the risk of breast cancer proportionally, and that the most frequent users (women given between twenty-six and fifty antibiotic prescriptions) had more than double the risk of breast cancer compared to women in the control group.

Antibiotics are one of the most common medications taken by pregnant women, and a new study has made convincing connections between antibiotic use during pregnancy and incidence of birth defects. Women who took sulfonamides and nitrofurantoins (frequently used for urinary tract infections) while pregnant were two to four times as likely to give birth to babies with heart defects.[9] The more commonly used penicillins, erythromycins, and cephalosporins were also each associated with at least one birth defect. It is also known that giving infants antibiotics in their first year of life triggers asthma and allergies that develop later on in childhood.[10] Yet more than half of all babies are given prescriptions for antibiotics before they turn one!

Antibiotics are risky medications that should be reserved for severe (and carefully documented) bacterial infections—infections that would seriously threaten the health of the patient if left untreated. We have powerful immune systems that, when supported by excellent nutrition, will clear the more moderate infections without help from drugs. (And don't miss the big-picture point: although most antibiotics are prescribed and taken for inappropriate indications, even the *appropriate* indications would not likely have occurred if superior nutrition and the resultant increased immunity to infection had been in place.)

The risks of antibiotics include diarrhea, digestive disturbances, yeast overgrowth, bone marrow suppression, seizures, kidney damage, severe bloody colitis, and life-threatening allergic reactions. In addition, in every single person who takes an antibiotic, the drug kills a broad assortment of helpful bacteria that live in the digestive tract and aid digestion. It kills the "bad" bacteria—such as those that can complicate an infection—but it also kills these helpful "good" bacteria lining your digestive tract that have properties protecting you from future illness. These changes in bacterial balance can take over a year to recover from after one course of antibiotics.

These are all individual consequences, but there are societal consequences as well. The overuse of antibiotics during past decades has been blamed for the recent emergence of antibiotic-resistant strains of deadly bacteria. By overprescribing antibiotics when they *aren't* needed, we have made these drugs less effective when they *are* needed.

The facts are documented, and yet too many of us remain unaware of the dangers of antibiotics—or are aware but remain unconcerned.

In the following pages, I will go through the various medical and non-medical remedies for colds and influenza and explain what works and what doesn't. There are a lot of myths and theories circulating.

But as you will continue to discover, we don't need to be on a roller coaster with our health. Creating Super Immunity will help prevent colds and influenza from occurring in the first place; and in the very rare circumstance that you do get sick, my approach will have you feeling yourself in no time. There are real, proven remedies available to you.

Healthy Bacteria

Given people's general willingness to take antibiotics at the drop of a hat, let's take a brief detour into the subject of healthy bacteria. Knowing the facts might make you less willing to take medications that target bacteria indiscriminately.

More than one-third of the dry weight of human stool is bacteria—bacteria that have been busily doing their job of food processing. Hundreds of different species of "good" bacteria play a very important role in our health; among other things, they process fiber and produce certain vitamins (such as B vitamins and vitamin K) and other nutritive substances. The health-promoting bacteria, called "probiotics," are normal inhabitants of the human gastrointestinal tract. Amazingly, bowel bacteria cells comprise approximately 95 percent of the total number of cells in the human body. These bowel inhabitants play a critical role in the health of our immune system.

Seventy percent of the immune system is located in the gastrointestinal (GI) tract, and the microflora (the bacterial population) of the GI tract constitute a complex ecosystem that can be viewed as an organ of the body. These microbes profoundly influence our health and survival. Certain normal metabolic functions and enzyme activities can be attributed to the microflora, which play a role in metabolizing nutrients, vitamins, drugs, endogenous hormones, and carcinogens; synthesizing fatty acids; preventing colonization of pathogens; and modulating the normal immune response.

For instance, these friendly flora make short-chain fatty acids (such as lipoic acid and butyrate) and other nutrients that have antioxidant and immune-enhancing properties. In addition to these health-enhancing activities that enable your body to function more efficiently, good intestinal bacteria secrete antibacterial substances that prevent *disease-causing* bacteria from taking hold in your body. In other words, the health-promoting bacteria crowd out and prevent the development of pathogens looking to take hold as bacterial illnesses. Having a proliferation of health-promoting bacteria is also thought to offer protection against colon cancer.

When you eat a healthy, micronutrient-rich, plant-based diet, you promote the growth of the *good* species of bacteria. The typical American (unhealthy) diet is lacking in these very powerful and protective bacteria and in fact promotes the growth of microbes that can damage your health and body.

If you take antibiotics repeatedly, you further diminish the population of good bacteria that protect you against the "harmful" bacteria. In addition, the "harmful" bacteria become more resistant (that is, harder to kill with antibiotics the next time). Over a hundred different helpful intestinal bacteria are lost with the use of antibiotics, which then gives disease-causing microbes the chance to proliferate and fill the ecological vacuum created by the repeated administration of antibiotics.

Here are the most important functions of intestinal microflora (good bacteria):

1. Supplement the digestive process to break down food

2. Produce vitamins, short-chain fatty acids, and proteins utilized by the body

3. Protect against the overgrowth of pathogenic bacteria and yeasts

4. Strengthen immune function

5. Create beneficial nutrients that prevent weight gain

Here, on the other hand, are the harmful effects of pathogenic bacteria and yeasts—those that can invade us if our population of *good* bacteria gets too low:

1. Produce toxic substances, including carcinogens

2. Harbor a reservoir of bacterial invaders to create future serious infections

3. Produce digestive disturbances

4. Promote immune system dysfunction and autoimmune inflammatory diseases

5. Promote weight gain

Anyone who pays attention to health news knows that deadly bacteria are a growing threat to everyone. Hardly a week goes by without an antibiotic-resistant bacteria turning up and threatening a community. Over a hundred thousand people die each year of hospital-acquired antibiotic-resistant infections.

As mentioned earlier, antibiotics are part of this problem. They cause bacteria to mutate relatively quickly to develop resistance. These resistant bacteria can then transfer genetic material to nonresistant bacteria, causing them, too, to become resistant.

Let's look at how this resistance comes about. Exposure to antibiotics kills off susceptible bacteria, but some *not* susceptible forms survive and then replicate in high numbers. As they replicate, part of their gene sequence, including information about how they defeated a particular antibiotic, gets spread into the surrounding area. Bacteria can even carry *multiple* gene sequences, offering resistance to a number of different bacteria. These resistant genes are then excreted by the bacteria in packages called "plasmids" and picked up by other bacteria. It is as if other bacteria were being inoculated with protection from antibiotics, thereby building and spreading superbugs that outwit drug use.

Repeated use of antibiotics over time can set the stage for recurrent infections and turn what might have started out as a minor illness into a more serious disease with a virulent bacteria at a later date. If you take antibiotics when they are not indicated, you increase the likelihood that you will develop an infection later on when they will be necessary. The problem is that at that point, if an antibiotic is truly needed for a potentially life-threatening infection such as a bacterial pneumonia, there is a higher probability that it simply won't work.

People die daily from infections that would have been easily treated by antibiotics in the past. Today microbes are resistant mostly as a result of the indiscriminate use of antibiotics for viral illnesses. The proper use of antibiotics for serious bacterial infections is actually relatively rare compared to the improper use for viral infections when they are not indicated. Later, we will review when antibiotics are appropriate and should be used with a bacterial infection. Just remember that this occurrence is extremely rare.

Before moving on to reviews of current cold and flu remedies, it is important that we stop and evaluate the good news. We have well within our reach the ability to stay healthy. With the right choices, we can radically improve our immune systems. We can start today with nearly immediate, profound, and long-lasting effects.

Common Cold and Flu Remedies

Many people ill with a cold, bronchitis (bad cold with cough), sinusitis (bad cold with stuffed face), or pharyngitis (bad cold with sore throat), will look for over-the-counter pharmaceutical products or alternative remedies for relief. Plus, using a scientific-sounding medical term such as sinusitis or bronchitis does not justify using antibiotics and other drugs. They are still viral illnesses.

Plus, most of the options that offer a degree of symptomatic relief have risks and toxicities that make the marginal amount of aid they offer not worth it. Treatments focus on relieving symptoms (e.g., cough, nasal congestion), but as symptoms are lessened, the person stays ill longer. Over-the-counter cold and flu remedies are also ineffective (or reduce symptoms only very temporarily) and are not without significant risk.

The symptoms we experience with illness are the body's natural healing and protective measures. Suppressing these more often than not extends the length of an illness. This is true with fever reducers, decongestants, cough suppressants, and similar remedies.

So how do we relieve these symptoms? We don't; instead, we provide our body the necessary ingredients to do its job. This means getting extra rest, eating well, and letting the body carry out its immune functions without interference.

Listed below are some of the most common treatments for colds and flu, along with both their intended effects and their side effects:

Cough Medications

Dextromethorphan is a popular cough suppressant. It is the active ingredient in many over-the-counter cold and cough remedies, such as NyQuil, Robitussin, Dimetapp, and others. Despite its wide use, it is not effective. In fact, a recent placebo-controlled trial in children demonstrated that those given the medication at night did not cough less, and they actually slept worse because of insomnia induced by the medication.[11]

Codeine has not been shown to effectively treat a cough caused by the common cold either. Although hydrocodone, a narcotic, is widely used and has been shown to be a mildly effectively cough suppressant, it has not been adequately evaluated in colds and has potentially serious side effects.

I was taught in medical school that it's a good thing these cough suppressants don't work, because if they did people would be in trouble.

As we touched on earlier, cough symptoms are there for a reason: to upwardly mobilize the mucous, dead cells, and virus particles and prevent that mucous from settling down and plugging the airways. If cough suppressants were effective and truly interrupted that cough function, viral illnesses would turn into more prolonged and serious illnesses, such as bacterial pneumonias.

Antihistamines

A Cochrane analysis of thirty-five controlled trials of antihistamines for colds and viral illness showed no evidence of significant improvement in the common cold; however, antihistamines did increase sleepiness.[12]

Antihistamines, combination antihistamine/decongestant therapies, and even topical nasal sprays can modestly improve symptoms in adults; however, they do not enable a faster recovery, and the very slight benefits must be weighed against potential side effects.[13] Common side effects include headache, stomach upset, constipation, rapid heartbeat, weakness, dizziness, difficulty urinating, trouble breathing, and even anxiety. Many consumers assume these side effects to be from the infection, not recognizing them as drug-induced. Newer nonsedating antihistamines, designed to minimize that particular side effect, are likewise ineffective against a cough.

I would recommend using antihistamines only if you are uncomfortably awake at night and unable to sleep.

Ibuprofen (Motrin and Advil) and Aspirin

In general, medications may relieve a small amount of discomfort from fever but do not enhance recovery. In fact, taking medications to reduce fever may actually prolong the illness.[14] Fever is a good thing when we have viral illnesses, as well as all infections, because it increases the ability of the white blood cells to sop up and kill viruses and virus-infected cells. Fever is a positive sign that the body is fighting the infection. When we suppress fevers with medication, we counter our body's ability to fight the illness. In fact, in animal studies, as temperature goes up, viral "load" comes down. Treatment with antipyretics (fever reducers) also prolongs viral "shedding," meaning that we are contagious, potentially passing the illness on to others, for a longer period.[15] Most important, according to a double-blind, placebo-controlled trial, the more we take these drugs, the worse we get and the longer we remain ill.[16] The use of aspirin and acetaminophen was associated with suppression of neutralizing antibody response and increased nasal symptoms and signs.

Certainly some ibuprofen at night, if discomfort is limiting sleep, may be appropriate, but it should be used sparingly.

AMERICAN ACADEMY OF PEDIATRICS (AAP): *AVOID* FEVER-REDUCING DRUGS

The AAP does not recommend treating your child with antipyretics (fever-reducing drugs), even with higher temperatures. As their website states:

> Fevers generally do not need to be treated with medication unless your child is uncomfortable or has a history of febrile convulsions. The fever may be important in helping your child fight the infection. Even higher temperatures are not in themselves dangerous or significant unless your child has a history of seizures or a chronic disease. Even if your child has a history of a fever-related convulsion and you treat the fever with medication, they may still have this kind of seizure. . . . If he is eating and sleeping well and has periods of playfulness, he probably doesn't need any treatment.

Acetaminophen (Tylenol)

Acetaminophen is more toxic than ibuprofen and is effective for only four to five hours anyway. It can cause liver damage even if taken in the recommended dosages, though in most of the documented cases of liver failure and death it was given or taken in a mistakenly elevated dose. In a person who is not eating or is vomiting or is dehydrated from illness, it can dramatically increase the potential for liver toxicity.

Acetaminophen is a significant cause of death in children, in part because it is such a common ingredient in fruity-tasting cold remedies. Children who help themselves to some extra cold medicine can put themselves in the danger zone. The risk of acetaminophen overdose in infants and children is exacerbated by the variable dosing schedules and the variety of formulations in the different products available. Many caring parents have unknowingly overmedicated their children, sometimes causing death, because they did not understand or follow the dosage recommendations.

In healthy adults, even a dose of 4 grams daily (the equivalent, typically, of eight extrastrength tablets) can cause liver function abnormalities; and lower, more standard dosages can cause digestive tract problems. Acetaminophen has also been shown to increase the risk of major cardiovascular events: heart attacks, congestive heart failure, and strokes. All patients, and particularly the parents of children, should be warned about acetaminophen use and taught about the serious risks associated with its use and overuse. For a drug with such potential toxicity, there is no reason to have it in the home.

Chicken Soup

Chicken soup has almost no effect on the common cold or other viral infections; however, eating lots of hot soup may temporarily lessen nasal symptoms. It certainly does not shorten the duration of infection, and in fact may even lengthen it via suppression of mucosal flow and white blood cell movement.[17]

Overall, the important point regarding eating when ill is to eat lightly and avoid animal products (like chicken) that are more demanding to digest. In other words, make it vegetable soup over chicken soup. (See soup recipes beginning on page 214.)

Humidified Air or Steam Inhalation

Using a vaporizer or humidifier likewise has little or no effect on recovery from illness. Studies have shown that it has no effect on wheezing or coughing in croup, or on resolution of symptoms or accelerating recovery in the common cold.[18]

Increased Intake of Fluids

"Drink plenty of fluids" is well-worn advice that is almost universally promoted by health professionals and family during illnesses. Surprisingly (given its pervasiveness), it has no basis in science. Certainly, dehydration can dry the respiratory mucosal surfaces and is important to prevent, especially when water losses occur from diarrhea, vomiting, and high fever. However, *excess* fluids (beyond replacement of losses) have no favorable benefits; there is no evidence that drowning in extra fluids improves resistance to viral infections or speeds recovery.

In short, there is currently no scientific evidence for increasing fluids in acute respiratory infections over and above the demands of thirst. On the contrary, some nonexperimental (observational) studies report that increasing fluid intake in acute respiratory infections may cause harm.[19] Outside of when it is replacing a loss of fluids, excess water consumption can have significant negative consequences. The key here is not to overly tax our body by asking it to do more than necessary.

Nasal Saline Irrigation

Flushing the sinuses daily with salty water may improve symptoms somewhat in people with chronic sinus infections,[20] but an analysis of all the studies done on this therapy for acute viral infections and the common cold shows no difference between treatment and controls.[21] That means subjecting your child to the discomfort of squirting water in his nose will not lessen complications or speed resolution of symptoms.

Homeopathic Remedies

Homeopathy (or homeopathic medicine) was developed in Germany more than two hundred years ago. The central homeopathic principle is that of "similars"—or "like cures like"—meaning that a disease can be cured by a toxic substance that produces symptoms similar to those of the disease or condition. Once a "similar" has been identified, it is diluted down so that scarcely any of the original substance can be detected in the product that is given as medication. Some believe that it is the "vibrational memory" of that substance that has healing properties.

Homeopathy was developed based on theories that are not consistent with accepted modern tenets of chemistry and physics. We also have greater understanding of the so-called placebo effect today and realize how important it is to do double-blind studies when evaluating the efficacy of treatments.

Today the word "homeopathic" is used as a marketing tool to sell herbal and nutritional products that have no resemblance to traditional homeopathic principles. In health food stores, it has turned into a marketing term without real meaning.

A number of bonafide homeopathic remedies are marketed as cold and flu products. Oscillococcinum is among the most popular products marketed for this purpose. A 2006 Cochrane review of this remedy, including three prevention trials and four treatment trials, concluded that it was not effective in preventing infections and had an insignificant effect on the duration of symptoms.[22]

Vitamin C

The role of vitamin C (ascorbic acid) in the prevention and treatment of the common cold has been a subject of controversy for sixty years, but vitamin C is still widely sold and used as both a preventive and a therapeutic agent. A Cochrane systematic review of thirty randomized trials involving more than 11,000 adults concluded that prophylactic vitamin C supplementation (200 milligrams or more daily) is not effective in reducing the incidence of upper-respiratory-tract infections in most adults.

While Vitamin C doesn't reduce the incidence of the common cold in the general population, it may be of some value in a select population with inadequate nutrition or under significant stress. In other words, for those who have inadequate consumption of raw fruits and vegetables (and therefore low levels of vitamin C and other antioxidants and immune-supporting phytochemicals), taking vitamin C may have some protective benefit, especially when those people are under physical or emotional stress; for those who already consume adequate vitamin C through raw fruits and vegetables, taking extra will have no advantage.

Once you are already sick, vitamin C has not been shown to be effective either. In the Cochrane meta-analysis that pooled together numerous studies on this subject, vitamin C demonstrated no benefits compared to placebos when taken at the onset of symptoms.[23] Likewise, no benefits were noted in the number of sick days or severity of symptoms.

My take on preventive vitamin C in the undernourished is clear—change to a diet rich in vitamin C and other beneficial nutrients and don't waste your money on supplemental vitamin C. Some nutritional supplements containing vitamins and herbs are marketed as cold fighters. Don't be taken in. Lawsuits for false advertising have ensued because the manufacturers make claims without real data to support their products' efficacy. Keep yourself healthy and disease-resistant all the time, so you don't have to look for magic when you get ill.

Echinacea

Echinacea used in children or adults has been investigated in a significant number of studies and has not been shown to be effective in lessening cold symptoms or shortening the length of illness.[24] In some of the studies, this herbal remedy seemed to have a significant benefit in reducing the incidence of viral infections when taken throughout the whole winter, but this result was not consistent among the better-quality, larger studies. This potential benefit may be less valid than reported.[25] Certainly, echinacea is not a major cornerstone of improving immunity against infections, though it can be used preventively throughout the winter cold and flu season.

Likewise, other herbs that are often recommended to treat viral infections—such as andrographis, ginseng, astragalus, golden seal, juniper, and pelargonium—may also have mild immune-stimulating effects or mild antihistaminic effects to lessen symptoms. However, the limited data that is available does not support a major shortening of the disease process or offer a major resistance to infection.

Most natural or folk remedies have not been tested in rigorous controlled trials; and for those that have, studies have often had mixed results. Be cautious, and please don't overuse any of the above.

Garlic

Garlic is a commonly used food and folk remedy for preventing and treating colds. However, there is still insufficient clinical trial evidence regarding the effectiveness of garlic in prevention or treatment. A single trial suggests that garlic may prevent occurrences of the common cold, but more studies are needed to validate this finding. Other studies haven't shown effectiveness of garlic as a treatment for the common cold, and claims of effectiveness appear to rely largely on poor-quality evidence.[26]

That doesn't mean garlic isn't useful. As we saw earlier, both garlic and onions are immune-enhancing foods. They may not rapidly change your immune function—not quickly enough to make a difference once you've become ill—but eating this family of foods on a regular basis is one of the components of Super Immunity.

My advice: continue to eat onions and garlic throughout the year and throughout any illness.

Resveratrol

The phytochemical compound resveratrol, found in the skin of red grapes, in berries, and in peanuts, appears to suppress inflammation and may fight aging in humans; however, long-term clinical trials in humans have not yet documented its benefits.

There *has* been research on this popular plant extract with *non*human subjects. Resveratrol has been shown to prolong life and reduce the rate of aging in worms, fruit flies, and yeast. In rodent studies it has been shown to have anticancer benefits.[27] It has also been shown to have antiproliferative effects on human cancer cells, and in a human controlled trial it was shown to decrease inflammatory markers after a high-fat meal.[28] Though this and other studies seem promising in terms of the potential anti-aging benefits of this compound in humans, we don't know whether a concentrated extract of resveratrol as a supplement is likely to be as helpful as the data from insect and animal studies suggests. Nevertheless, the data collected so far is promising.

Furthermore, resveratrol seems to have broad antiviral effects. The rodent studies (while not high-quality, controlled human clinical trials) are nevertheless impressive. Studies show that resveratrol inhibits replication of herpes simplex virus (HSV) types 1 and 2 at an early step in the virus replication cycle. Studies in mice also show that resveratrol inhibits or reduces HSV replication in the vagina and inhibits varicella-zoster virus and influenza virus, and enhances the anti-HIV-1 activity of several anti-HIV drugs.

My recommendation here is cautious, but hopeful. Since resveratrol and its related compounds have so many potentially beneficial properties and protect against and fight cancer from so many angles, from angiogenesis inhibition to preventing tumor initiation by deactivating carcinogens,[29] I think it likely that supplementing with resveratrol is beneficial; resveratrol may turn out to be an important adjunct, not just preventatively but also for patients who already are diagnosed with cancer. Eating colorful fruits and berries regularly gives us this compound.

If you are immune-challenged or susceptible to infections, consider a resveratrol supplement on a regular basis.

Zinc

Zinc, an essential mineral that plays an important role in immune function, is a nutrient that many people are borderline deficient in. The RDI (recommended daily intake) for zinc is 15 milligrams a day, a quantity not usually achieved by those not taking supplements or eating foods fortified with zinc—especially vegans, vegetarians, or flexitarians not eating seafood and meat daily.

Zinc deficiency leads to dysfunction of both antibody-mediated (humoral) and cell-mediated immunity and thus increases susceptibility to infection. There is considerable evidence to suggest that regular supplementation with zinc or deliberate consumption of foods rich in zinc is useful to improve immune function and fight off both infections and cancer.

Studies have been consistently positive in demonstrating that zinc deficiency is associated with an increased incidence and severity of infections and that zinc supplementation is beneficial.

- Zinc supplementation decreases incidence of pneumonia and antibiotic use.[30]

- Zinc supplementation decreases the duration of colds and flu by a day or more.

- Maternal zinc supplementation leads to a decrease in infant infections.

- Zinc supplementation decreases child mortality by more than 50 percent.[31]

The largest and most conclusive analysis of this issue (the respected Cochrane meta-analysis) concluded that once a person had a cold or flu, zinc supplements significantly reduced the severity of cold symptoms as well as the length of illness.[32] Among people taking zinc within twenty-four hours of the start of symptoms, the risk of still having symptoms at the seven-day mark was about half that of those not taking zinc. The review found that not only did zinc reduce the duration and severity of common cold symptoms, but regular zinc use also worked to prevent colds, leading to fewer school absences and less antibiotic use in children. In preventing colds, zinc supplements taken for at least five months reduced the risk of catching a cold to only two-thirds that of people not taking the supplements.

FOODS RICH IN ZINC

Oysters, farmed, eastern, cooked, 3 medium—13 mg

Alaska king crab, cooked, 1 leg—10.2 mg

Beef, top sirloin, 4 oz—5.6 mg

Raw, unhulled sesame seeds, 2 oz—4.4 mg

Raw or roasted pumpkin seeds, 2 oz—4.2 mg

Adzuki beans, cooked, 1 cup—4.1 mg

Raw pine nuts, 2 oz—3.6 mg

Raw cashews, 2 oz—3.2 mg

Sunflower seeds, raw, 2 oz—2.8 mg

Wild rice, cooked, 1 cup—2.2 mg

Edamame, cooked, shelled, 1 cup—2.1 mg

Black beans, kidney beans, cooked, 1 cup—1.9 mg

Shiitake mushrooms, cooked, 1 cup—1.9 mg

Fava beans, cooked, 1 cup—1.7 mg

Broccoli, cooked, 2 cups—1.6 mg

Tahini, raw, 2 tbsp—1.4 mg

Kale, cooked, 2 cups—1.2 mg

Overall, then, it seems prudent to avoid zinc deficiency and regularly supplement with zinc, with the caveat that zinc supplementation, whether throughout the year or only when ill, is not likely to be effective for well-nourished populations with excellent zinc stores already.

Those on vegetarian-style diets that are not ideally designed to include sufficient seeds and beans, and those on diets with low calorie intake, should consider taking a zinc supplement on a regular basis (if it is not in the multi you're already taking).

Vitamin D

Vitamin D is unique: it is more like a hormone than a vitamin and is not readily found in our food supply. That's why it is often called the sunshine vitamin. It has been suspected for centuries that declining sunlight during winter months could be a factor promoting increases in infections including influenza during the winter. A study done in 2006 with children who were given vitamin D and exposed to the influenza virus documented a reduced incidence of viral respiratory infections in the wintertime.[33] This suggests that vitamin D sufficiency may reduce infection to viruses via its ability to modulate the immune system, increasing the effectiveness of major immunity players, including macrophages, neutrophils, monocytes, and natural killer cells. These results have been supported by other studies that show an increased risk for acute lower-respiratory illness in people with low vitamin D levels; additionally, vitamin D deficiency has been associated with an increased risk for influenza.[34] Clearly, it is prudent to avoid vitamin D insufficiency. Maintaining adequate levels of vitamin D year-round is an important part of achieving Super Immunity.

Elderberry Extract

Black elderberry juice is widely used to treat colds and the flu. Studies suggest that black elderberry extract (2–3 tablespoons daily for adults and 1–4 teaspoons for children, depending on age) can inhibit the growth of influenza viruses and shorten the duration of influenza symptoms, while enhancing antibody levels against the virus.[35] Even though the studies are preliminary, the evidence suggests that these berries have beneficial properties to enhance the body's defense against viral infections, particularly influenza.[36]

The main flavonoids present in elderberries are the anthocyanins; cyanidin 3-glucoside and cyanidin 3-sambubioside have been identified to increase the defensive function of monocytes against viral-infected cells. More interestingly, elderberry has been demonstrated to inhibit the adhesion of the virus to the cell receptors. When the virus is inhibited from entering cells, it cannot replicate itself, and this can lessen the seriousness of the infection.

Anthocyanins are colored red, purple, black, or blue and are found in berries, eggplant skins, currant and grape skins, cherries, and black rice. Anthocyanins also account for the therapeutic potential of tart cherry juice, which is helpful for inflammatory conditions for the same reason. The small bluish-blackish elderberry is not a sweet-tasting fruit, but when you concentrate it as a liquid syrup or juice, you get a high concentration of these colorful pigments, making absorption more significant than from plain berries. This is one of the few remedies that is safe and very likely has some efficacy without being toxic.

Reviewing Recommendations for Preventing/Treating Illness

The bottom line is that while powdered fruit and vegetable supplements,[37] multivitamins,[38] and other health remedies—even garlic and vitamin C or E—may show some benefits in those with deficient or marginal intake of antioxidants and phytochemicals, the best and most effective way to prevent illness is with comprehensive nutritional adequacy maintained all year (following the dietary and supplemental recommendations contained within this book). An improved diet is more effective than any of these specific cold remedies.

Almost every family has their favored remedies and advice. From eating chicken soup, to wearing cloves of garlic around the neck, to wearing warm hats, you probably learned your immunity-enhancing ideas from your mother, who learned them from *her* mother. Unfortunately, chicken soup, steam vaporizers, hot tea with honey, and smelly salves on the chest have no scientific data to document effectiveness; most, in fact, have mostly been debunked in scientific investigations. When scrutinized via high-quality placebo trials, almost all remedies have shown no significant *treatment* effects (except in people who were somewhat nutritionally deficient). For example, pomegranate is a super food that builds stronger immune function, and the long-term use of it and other highly nutritious super foods may decrease incidence of infections—in other words, these foods help with *prevention*. However, pomegranate and the other super foods should not be seen as cold remedies. Rather, these highly nutritious foods support a normally functioning immune system.

Even vitamin D, elderberry, and zinc, with *proven* efficacy, are likely of value only in people whose levels are suboptimal. The goal, then, is still to achieve nutritional adequacy and forget the idea of nutritional remedies when ill. Take 15 milligrams of zinc per day all year, increasing that to 30 milligrams with the onset of cold symptoms. Probiotics and elderberry syrup are likely worth a try when you're ill. (Let me know if you think they worked for you.)

Let's review our findings:

A Likely Waste of Your Time	Likely Helpful
Vitamin C	
Chicken soup	Zinc
Humidified air	Vitamin D
Nasal saline irrigation	Elderberry and berry flavonoids
Echinacea	Caloric restriction

Finally, remember these important points when ill:

1. The greenish or yellow color of respiratory mucous does not mean you have a bacterial infection.

2. Expectorants and cough suppressants do not work and will not facilitate your recovery.

3. Neither taking vitamin C nor pushing fluids is useful.

4. Humidifiers and steam showers are not effective either.

5. Cool baths for lowering the fever should be avoided; they do not keep the fever down for long, and the fever itself heightens the effectiveness of the immune attack.

6. Avoid acetaminophen and other fever reducers; if you are too uncomfortable to sleep at night, take ibuprofen with some food.

7. If significantly ill, watch for the signs that a medical consultation is indicated (see chapter 2).

8. Reduce food intake and consume primarily vegetable juice, vegetable soup, water, and raw salad vegetables.

So now that we know what works and what doesn't work when it comes to colds and flu, let's return to our diet and check out the best healthy fats, carbohydrates, and proteins. You might just be surprised by what you will discover.

CHAPTER FIVE

Healthy Carbs, Fats, and Proteins

The most consistent and proven concept in the history of nutritional science is that the combination of high-nutrient intake and low-caloric intake promotes disease resistance and longevity. It is the basis for my health equation:

$$Health = Nutrients/Calories$$

What this equation means is that your health will improve as you eat more foods with a *high* nutrient-per-calorie density and fewer foods with a *low* nutrient-per-calorie density. First and foremost, avoid low-nutrient foods such as white breads and processed foods. White flour, other refined grains (such as those found in sweetened breakfast cereals), soft drinks, sweets, and even fruit juices are weight-promoting, lead to diabetes, and raise triglyceride and cholesterol levels, increasing heart attack risk. Furthermore, these low-nutrient processed foods also suppress immune function, increasing one's risk of infection and cancer. Incredibly, by 2010 these processed foods had become 62 percent of the calories in the standard American diet.

Consuming calories without the beneficial presence of antioxidants, vitamins, and phytochemicals leads to a buildup of waste products in the cells. When you eat white bread or other processed foods without enough accompanying plant-derived micronutrients, the body can't remove normal cellular wastes. When our cells don't have the raw materials needed for normal function, we age prematurely and become susceptible to disease.

The three macronutrients—fat, carbohydrate, and protein—supply us with calories. Certainly Americans eat too many calories, but there is no health advantage in making your diet extremely low in fat. I intentionally do not give a specific percentage of each macronutrient in the diet, and I do not recommend that fat be avoided. Trying to micromanage the precise amount of each caloric source misses the most critical issue in human nutrition.

The essential issue in human nutrition is meeting your *macro*nutrient needs without excess calories, and getting sufficient *micro*nutrients in the process. There is a broad acceptable range in the macronutrient ratio, as long as one is not overeating calories and one's body fat percentage is favorable. You may be surprised to learn that adhering to a diet that is *less* than 10 percent of calories from fat is *not* an appropriate recommendation for ideal health, and indeed often results in less than ideal health outcomes. However, one could be on a healthy diet that is 15 percent of calories from fat, or a healthy diet that is 30 percent of calories from fat. As long as the diet is rich in micronutrients and does not exceed our need for calories, the lower-fat diet has no advantage in the prevention and treatment of disease.

There is no evidence to suggest that a diet of equal calories that is lower in fat is an advantage for prevention or treatment of heart disease or any other disease. Studies that compare dietary fat percentages suggest that it is not the fat level but other more critical qualities that make the diet more or less beneficial.

While the fat percentage does not determine the quality of your diet, the amount of colorful vegetables does. To achieve an ideal level of phytonutrients and other micronutrients, you have to eat a large amount of green vegetables each day. Generally speaking, you can rate the nutritional quality of a diet by the percentage of colorful vegetables it contains. When you eat lots of vegetables, especially green vegetables, you meet your body's need for fiber and micronutrients with very few calories. Then, to comprise the balance of the diet and fill your caloric needs, you can choose an assortment of other foods, preferably including other foods with a decent micronutrient load. So when you eat more greens and other colorful vegetables and more fruits, beans, nuts, and seeds, you naturally eat less of other foods of a lower nutritional quality; that means fewer animal products and processed foods but also less oil, white bread, potato, and rice.

With that general grounding, let's now look at carbs, fats, and proteins in more detail.

All Carbohydrates Are Not Equal

Certainly most of us understand that a wild blueberry, strawberry, or cauliflower floret is a nutrient-rich source of carbohydrate, especially when compared to a candy bar or a slice of white bread. Not only do the natural, healthy carbohydrate foods contain more micronutrients, but they are also loaded with fiber and so-called resistant starch, both of which keep these foods' glycemic index (an index of their rate of conversion to sugar) and caloric density low. Resistant starch is like fiber in that it is resistant to digestion and does not break down to glucose or other simple sugars. It is a "prebiotic," something that promotes the growth of beneficial bacteria, or probiotics, in the digestive tract; these bacteria then break down the resistant starch into favorable compounds that improve our immune system function and reduce cancer risk.[1]

So the healthiest starches are in high-fiber, natural foods. These are typically low in absorbable calories, and they give us lots of micronutrients per caloric buck—not just an injection of glucose into our system.

The aforementioned glycemic index (GI) evaluates the blood glucose response in a fixed amount of carbohydrate in particular foods on a scale of 1 to 100. Glycemic load (GL) is a similar ranking, but it is generally thought to be more meaningful because it takes into account the carbohydrate content of a certain portion size of each food rather than a fixed number of grams of carbohydrate. Diets containing large quantities of high-GL foods are associated with the risk of diabetes, heart disease, multiple cancers, and overall chronic disease.[2] That means a

GLYCEMIC INDEX (GI) AND GLYCEMIC LOAD (GL) OF COMMON PLANT FOODS*

FOOD	GI	GL
Black beans	30	7
Red kidney beans	25	8
Lentils	30	5
Split peas	25	6
Black-eyed peas	30	13
Corn	52	9
Barley	35	16
Brown rice	75	18
Millet	71	25
Rolled oats	55	13
White rice	83	23
Whole wheat	70	14
White pasta	55	23
Sweet potato	61	17
White potato	(average) 90	26

* Foster-Powell K, Holt SHA, Brand-Miller JC. International table of glycemic index and glycemic load values: 2002. Am J Clin Nutr 2002;76:5–56.

diet with lots of bagels, cold cereals, pasta, white potatoes, and sweet desserts and snacks is not just fattening; it also promotes cancer. It's not that you cannot eat *any* high-GL foods; it's just that your diet should contain only a limited amount of those foods. Most of your carbohydrate intake should come from low-GL sources such as beans, vegetables, and berries.

There is a nutritional hierarchy of carbohydrate-rich plant foods. Beans, starchy vegetables, intact grains, and certain other nutritious natural foods are generally the most heavily emphasized in my recommendations, not just because of their favorable glycemic scores, but because they are richer in micronutrients, fiber, and resistant starch too. Interestingly, the micronutrient density of high-carb plant foods parallels their fiber and resistant starch content.

Regardless of the relative merits of these natural carbohydrates, things get considerably worse when they become processed. A perfect example is a cereal that consists of finely ground flour combined with fruit juice to sweeten it. When this processing occurs, it results in a food with a high glycemic effect and without significant micronutrient content.

Acceptable Carbohydrates

So what are the specific foods you want to include in your diet, to utilize the best high-carbohydrate foods? You've got a wide range of acceptable options.

Beans, peas, corn, wild rice, barley, steel-cut oats, oatmeal, tomatoes, squashes, berries, and fresh fruits are examples of the most favorable carbohydrates sources. Beans, green peas, berries, and tomatoes are at the top of the list. Squashes, intact whole grains (such as steel-cut oats), wild rice, quinoa, wheat berries, and even sweet potatoes would be more favorable choices than white potatoes, which would be at the bottom of this list.

Resistant Starch + Fiber in Common Plant Foods

RS = resistant starch   Percentages expressed as grams per 100 grams dry matter

FOOD	% RS	% FIBER	% RS + FIBER	DR. FUHRMAN'S NUTRIENT DENSITY SCORES
Black beans	26.9	42.6	69.5	10
Northern beans	28.0	41.1	69.1	11
Navy beans	25.9	36.2	62.1	8
Red kidney beans	24.6	36.8	61.4	11
Lentils	25.4	33.1	58.5	14
Split peas	24.5	33.1	57.6	7
Black-eyed peas	17.7	32.6	50.3	8
Corn	25.2	19.6	44.7	4
Barley	18.2	17.0	35.2	3
Brown rice	14.8	5.1	20.5	3
Millet	12.6	5.4	18.0	2
Rolled oats	7.2	10.0	17.2	2
White rice	14.1	1.5	15.6	1
Whole wheat	1.7	12.1	13.8	2
White pasta	3.3	5.6	8.9	1
Sweet potato	-	3.0	-	9
White potato	7.0	2.0	9.0	2

Unacceptable Carbohydrates

All of the above acceptable carbs are rendered unacceptable with excessive processing. In addition, you want to avoid the following:

Sweeteners, sugar, honey, maple syrup

White flour

White rice

Whole-grain pastry flour

Packaged cold cereals

Commercial fruit juices and even fruit-juice-sweetened beverages

Remember, high-glycemic, nutrient-sparse processed foods are not just fattening; they also suppress the immune system and increase the risk of cancer.[3] Most of us are unaware that croissants, white bread, bagels, pasta, cakes, cupcakes, pancakes, and most other "white" foods have been linked to many different types of cancer.

> A good rule is to avoid anything that is "white," such as sugar, white flour, white pasta, white potato, or white rice. Remember this rhyme: "The whiter the bread, the sooner you're dead."

Carbs as Just One Part of the Package

You shouldn't consider only the quality of your carbohydrate choices, of course, but the quality of your fat and protein choices as well. Though "carbs" is a popular buzzword these days, you want to consider what other beneficial nutrients come along for the ride in any food's natural package. It is the quality of the fat, the quality of the protein, and the quality of the carbohydrate you eat—in combination—that influences your health. Ask yourself, Is the food I am about to eat a whole, natural plant source of calories? Is it packaged with fiber, antioxidants, and phytochemicals? Does it contain not just discovered nutrients, but plenty of undiscovered nutrients too?

You will generally know the answers to these questions based on the degree of processing. Most of those fragile but beneficial nutrients are lost in foods that are heavily processed or prepared. These are the important issues to consider—far more important than whether a food is high or low in carbs, or high or low in fat or protein.

Fat: The Most Misunderstood Macronutrient

If you were to ask a hundred people which of the three macronutrients is the least necessary—indeed, the most harmful—chances are every one of them would name fat. And yet, as was noted in the introduction to this chapter, too *little* fat is a bad thing.

Fat Deficiency and Failure to Thrive

For many, an undue emphasis on extremely low-fat diets has resulted in health difficulties, and individuals following such recommendations have not thrived on a vegan or a flexitarian diet. Most often these individuals never realize what the problem is. They often go back to eating large amounts of animal products without discovering that some of the issues they experienced were due to fat deficiency on their low-fat diet.

Some of the health issues related to fat deficiency are dry skin, thinning hair, muscle cramps, poor sleep, high triglycerides, and poor exercise tolerance. For most fat-deficient individuals, eating more healthy fats, taking supplemental docosahexaenoic acid (DHA)—the long-chain omega-3 fat primarily responsible for the benefits of fish oil—and eating fewer processed foods and starchy carbohydrates clears up the problem. Some people simply require more essential fatty acids, period—both omega-6 and omega-3.

Insufficient fat in the diet can also compromise the absorption of fat-soluble vitamins and healthful phytochemicals. Seeds and nuts are the best high-fat foods. When you eat seeds and nuts with your meals, the fatty acids supplied increase the absorption of immune system–supporting micronutrients and phytochemicals significantly. For example, when you eat a nut- or seed-based dressing on a salad, you absorb much more of the carotenoids in the raw vegetables. More than ten times as much of certain nutrients is absorbed.

A study detecting blood levels of alpha-carotene, beta-carotene, and lycopene found negligible levels after ingestion of the salads with fat-free salad dressing, and high levels after the same foods were eaten with fatty dressings.[4]

As noted earlier, evidence has accumulated that a diet as low as 10 percent of calories from fat is too low—even for the overweight, diabetic, or heart disease patient. Judicious use of higher-fat foods is beneficial for not just heart disease, but weight loss and diabetes too. The scientific literature corroborates my clinical experience over the last fifteen years caring for thousands of patients with obesity, diabetes, cancer, and heart disease, and provides evidence to show that for every calorie removed from the diet from rice, potato, bread, or animal products and substituted with raw seeds and nuts, you get many health benefits, such as the following:[5]

- Lower blood sugar

- Lower cholesterol

- A better LDL/HDL cholesterol ratio

- Lower triglycerides

- Better antioxidant status

- Better absorption of phytochemicals from vegetables

- Better diabetic control

- Lower weight, not weight gain

- More effective reversal of heart disease

- Prevention of cardiac arrhythmias (in heart patients)

- Better nutritional diversity and satisfaction with fewer calories

- Increased protection against cancer

- Better muscle and bone mass with aging

Seeds and Nuts: An Undeserved Bad Rap

Raw nuts and seeds are packed with nutrients, as we saw in an earlier chapter. They contain lignans, bioflavonoids, minerals, and other antioxidants that protect the fragile freshness of the fats therein; and they contain plant proteins and plant sterols that naturally lower cholesterol. They also contain powerful ellagitannins (ETs). These dietary polyphenols with potent antioxidant and other cancer-preventive properties are found in berries, nuts, and seeds; they are best absorbed from walnuts.[6]

Nuts, seeds, and avocados are high-fat foods, yet evidence from many different studies shows a wide variety of health benefits from eating these foods.[7] It is important to emphasize that the health problems associated with a high-fat diet come from consuming animal fats, processed oils, and trans fats, not from the consumption of raw nuts and seeds. There has never been a study that showed any negative health outcome from consuming these natural, high-fat, whole plant foods. In fact, the studies all show positive health benefits and conclude that these foods should be an important part of a well-rounded diet.

Nuts and seeds average about 175 calories an ounce, and one or two ounces a day would consist of 15 to 30 percent of a daily caloric intake from the fat range. As an added benefit, the addition of seeds and nuts increases the plant protein in your diet. In other words, as you eat less animal protein and instead substitute more plant protein from nuts, seeds, beans, and greens, your nutrient levels skyrocket and your health improves.

The protective effect of nut consumption on heart disease is not offset by increased mortality from other causes. In other words, in all populations, sexes, and ages, as nut consumption increases, death from all causes decreases and overall lifespan increases as well.[8] Please note, though, that these powerful health benefits are *not* achieved when oils, rather than whole nuts and seeds, are substituted as a caloric source.

Misconceptions About Olive Oil

No oil should be considered a health food. All oil, including nut and olive oil, is 100 percent fat and contains 120 calories per tablespoon. Oil is high in calories, low in nutrients, and contains no fiber. Throw a few tablespoons of oil on your salad or vegetable dish and you've added hundreds of wasted calories. Simply put, it is the perfect food to help you put on unwanted and unhealthful pounds.

When you consume oil (*any* type of oil), there are no fat-binding fibers remaining from the original oil source. That means all the calories are absorbed rapidly and stored away as body fat within minutes. When you eat whole seeds and nuts, on the other hand, the fat is bound to sterols and stanols and other plant fibers. This binding of the fats in the digestive tract limits their absorption and actually attracts some of the negative fats circulating in the blood and draws them into the digestive tract for excretion in the stool. Put another way, the fats eaten intact in seeds and nuts are not all "biologically available." As a result, significant calories do not get absorbed, and therefore the seeds and nuts are not as fattening as the same amount of calories from oil would be; in addition, they contain numerous protective nutrients that are not in the oil.

Think about it: oil is a *processed* food. When you chemically extract oil from a whole food (such as olives, nuts, or seeds), you leave behind—lose!—the vast majority of micronutrients and end up with a fragmented food that contains little more than empty calories. When you consume whole foods such as walnuts, sesame seeds, and flax seeds instead of their extracted oils, you get all of the fibers, flavonoids, and nutrients they contain, as well as all of their positive health benefits.

It's true that foods rich in monounsaturated fats like olive oil are less harmful than foods full of saturated fats and trans fats. But being less harmful does not make them "healthful." The beneficial effects of the Mediterranean diet are not due to the consumption of olive oil;

they are due to antioxidant-rich foods, including vegetables, fruits, and beans. Eating a lot of any kind of oil means you're eating a lot of empty calories, which leads to excess weight and can also lead to diabetes, high blood pressure, stroke, heart disease, and many forms of cancer.

You can add a little bit of olive oil to your diet if you are thin and exercise a lot. However, the more oil you add, the more you are lowering the nutrient-per-calorie density of your diet—and that is *not* your objective, as it does not promote health.

Epidemiologic studies on nuts indicate an inverse association between frequency of consumption and weight, contrary to the situation with oil consumption. Although seeds and nuts are not low in calories and indeed are relatively high in fat, their consumption may actually suppress appetite and help people get rid of diabetes and lose weight.[9] In other words, people who consume more nuts and seeds are likely to be slim, and people consuming less of such foods are more likely to be heavier.

In well-controlled trials that looked to see if eating nuts and seeds resulted in weight gain, the results showed the opposite; eating raw nuts and seeds promoted weight *loss,* not weight *gain.* Several studies also have shown that eating a small amount of nuts or seeds helps dieters feel satiated, stay with the program, and have more success at long-term weight loss.[10]

Should we all sit in front of our TV, eat an entire bag of nuts in an hour, and complain when we gain weight? Of course not! Healthy eaters avoid excess calories and do not eat for recreation. Eat only an ounce of nuts a day if you are significantly overweight; but if you are thin, physically active, pregnant, or nursing, eat 2 to 4 ounces (according to your caloric needs).

Remember that when you eat these high-fat foods with your meals, they facilitate the absorption of beneficial phytochemicals from other foods. Save them to eat with your vegetable meals, and especially in salad dressings. Also, it is best to eat nuts and seeds raw or only lightly toasted. When you *roast* nuts and seeds, you form carcinogenic acrylamides as the food is browned, and you decrease the protein and create more ash from the roasting process. The more nuts and seeds are cooked, the more amino acids are destroyed. You also lower levels of calcium, iron, selenium, and other minerals in the roasting process.

The Protein Puzzle

Our entire society is on a protein binge, brainwashed with poor information. We need to separate fact from fiction so that we can determine which protein sources our bodies benefit from most.

Animal Protein vs. Plant-Based Protein

The nutrition-related educational materials used in most schools have been provided "gratis" by the meat, dairy, and egg industries for over seventy years. Those industries have successfully lobbied and influenced the government, resulting in favorable laws and subsidies—and resulting in advertising propaganda being fed to every child. They have been selling the mistaken idea that we need meat, dairy, and eggs in order to be properly nourished. We have thus been programmed with incorrect and dangerous information.

Almost all Americans get more than enough protein daily. In fact, the average American consumes over 100 grams of protein, about 50 percent more than the recommended daily amount. Yet too many of us, including athletes, fitness enthusiasts, bodybuilders, dieters, and the overweight, turn to protein powders, protein drinks, and nutrition bars in a quest for even more protein.

The overall goal is to eat fewer animal products in general so that we can reduce the amount of protein from animal sources and increase the amount of protein from plant sources.

It is true that a certain lifestyle, one involving vigorous and regular physical workouts, requires additional protein. For example, resistance training and endurance workouts can break down muscle protein and increase our need for protein to fuel repair and growth. But the increased need for protein is proportional to the increased need for extra calories burned from the exercise. As exercise increases our appetite, we increase our caloric intake accordingly—and our protein intake increases proportionally. If we meet the increased caloric demand from heavy exercise with an ordinary assortment of natural plant foods—vegetables, whole grains, beans, seeds, and nuts—we will get the precise amount of extra protein needed. A typical assortment of vegetables, nuts, seeds, beans, and whole grains supply about 50 grams of protein per 1000 calories. Don't forget, green vegetables are almost 50 percent protein, and when you eat more vegetables, it gives you your protein in a Super Immunity and anticancer package.

When the additional calories are derived from health-enhancing plant foods, you will get much more than just protein; these foods will supply you with a host of antioxidants to protect against the increased free radicals generated by the exercise. Nature planned this pretty well!

Take a look at this sampling of foods, shown with their caloric and protein content:

PROTEIN CONTENT OF COMMON PLANT FOODS

	CALORIES	PROTEIN IN GRAMS
One cup peas	120	9
One cup lentils	175	16
Two cups spinach	84	10.8
Two slices whole-grain bread	120	10
One ear corn on the cob	150	4.2
One cup brown rice	220	4.8
Two ounces sunflower seeds	175	7.5
TOTAL	1044	62.3

Consider that the maximum muscle mass the human body can typically add in one week is about one pound. That's the upper limit of the muscle fiber's capacity to make protein into muscle; any protein beyond that is simply converted to fat. Although athletes have a greater protein requirement than sedentary individuals, this extra is easily obtained through the diet; the use of protein supplements is not merely a waste of money, it is unhealthy.

Taking in more protein, especially animal protein, than your body needs is not a small matter. It ages you prematurely and can cause significant harm. The excess protein you are *not* using isn't stored by the body as protein; it is converted to fat, or it is eliminated via the kidneys. Eliminating excess nitrogen via the urine leaches calcium and other minerals from the bones and breeds kidney stones. Vegetable foods are alkaline. Animal products are acidic foods, and they require a huge output of hydrochloric acid from the stomach to digest them. This acid tide in the blood, after a high-protein meal, requires an equally strong base response by the body to neutralize the acid. We get the needed base contribution at the expense of our bones, which give up their minerals; our bones literally dissolve for that purpose into phosphates and calcium. This is a primary step in bone loss that leads to osteoporosis. Our high salt intake then further contributes to flushing our bone mass down the toilet bowl. The excessive stimulation of bone turnover also causes an increase in bone breakdown and remodeling, which can lead to osteoarthritis and calcium deposits in other tissues.

Exercise, not extra protein, builds strength, denser bones, and bigger muscles. When you artificially stimulate growth with overfeeding and excessive animal product consumption, you may achieve a heightened body mass index (a weight-to-height ratio), but this will add fat to your body as well. Let me caution you that a higher body mass index, even if that additional body mass is mostly muscle, is linked to an earlier death. Large football players have over twice the risk of early cardiac death than the general population, with many of them dying before their fiftieth birthday.[11] Out of more than six hundred Olympic athletes on the East German 1964 Olympic team, fewer than ten are still alive today. Promoting muscular growth with supplements and steroids doesn't seem too wise, when seen in that context. Excessive body mass, even excessive muscular development from overeating high-protein animal products, is a risk factor for heart attacks and other diseases later in life.

We can't judge health by size; we must judge it by resistance to serious illnesses, longevity potential, and maintaining our useful vigor and athleticism into our later years. When you're trying to exercise for health and eat for health, one of your goals should be to reduce rather than increase animal food consumption and animal-derived protein.

The Protein Paradox

A hormone known as "insulin-like growth factor 1" (IGF-1) is one of the body's important growth promoters in the womb and during childhood growth, but it also has some anabolic (or bodybuilding) effects in adulthood. A person's IGF-1 production is promoted by consuming more protein of a high biological value—which is to say, protein that contains all of the essential amino acids in the proportion that maximally promotes growth. The protein from animal products fits that description: it is of a very high biological value. Thus our society's mistaken preoccupation with maximizing size and growth through the high consumption of animal protein has driven up IGF-1 levels.

The production of IGF-1 takes place primarily in the liver, and its production is stimulated by something called "pituitary-derived growth hormone" (GH). IGF-1 is a key contributor to brain development, muscle and bone growth, and sexual maturation. The highest levels of IGF-1 occur during the growth spurt and the sexual maturation phase of puberty. The issue here is that *elevated* IGF-1 levels, resulting from today's animal-protein-heavy diet, have been linked to cancer; indeed, they are thought to bear considerable responsibility for the high rates of cancer in the modern world.

Scientists first noted that higher levels of sex hormones such as estrogen and testosterone were associated with breast cancer; more recently, insulin and IGF-1 have been demonstrated to be important promoters of cancer as well. The connection between increased IGF-1 and cancer has been recognized for many years. In fact, cancer drugs targeting the IGF-1 pathway began to be developed in the late 1990s, and over seventy clinical trials have begun since then, many with encouraging results.[12] Since IGF-1 plays a key role in tumor growth, reducing IGF-1 levels by dietary methods is now considered by scientists to be an effective cancer-prevention measure.

IGF-1 is crucial for growth and development in childhood, as noted earlier; but if levels remain high during adulthood, it speeds aging, reduces immune function, and promotes cancer. Conversely, reduced IGF-1 has been associated with enhanced lifespan.[13] Our nation's mistaken overemphasis on protein, with the resulting elevation of IGF-1 levels, has clearly played a destructive role in the exploding cancer epidemic of the last hundred years. Excess intake of refined carbohydrates can also have a detrimental effect on IGF-1 levels. The intake of those carbohydrates leads to an increase in the production of insulin, which regulates energy metabolism (while also increasing production of IGF-1 and decreasing production of IGF-binding proteins).[14] Type 2 diabetes, in which the body can't properly use what insulin there is, is associated with breast, colon, and pancreatic cancer, and there is evidence that insulin-mediated stimulation of IGF-1 production is partially responsible for this increase in cancer.[15]

Due to decreased secretion of growth hormone (GH), IGF-1 levels naturally decline with age. On average, serum IGF-1 is approximately 150 nanograms per milliliter at age fifty, and 100 nanograms per milliliter at age eighty.[16] Since GH can stimulate muscle growth, it used to be prescribed by some alternative-medicine physicians, who promoted it as an anti-aging hormone. However, studies found that restoring GH to youthful concentrations was not beneficial; in fact, GH treatment increased mortality in elderly and ill patients, and increased diabetes and glucose intolerance in healthy adults.

Today there is a tremendous amount of evidence regarding the lifespan-enhancing effects from *lowered* levels of IGF-1 in adulthood.[17] Not only do higher IGF-1 levels promote cancer, but they also increase potential for dementia. Elevated circulating IGF-1 levels have been found to promote Alzheimer's disease, and reduced IGF-1 has been found to reduce symptoms of neuro-degeneration.[18] In tissues that require IGF-1 for proper function in adulthood, "local" production of IGF-1 in exercised muscle tissues compensates for the lower circulating IGF-1 levels. In other words, lower levels are longevity-promoting and without apparent drawbacks.[19]

The body's cells are replicating all the time. As cell damage takes place, high circulating IGF-1 levels promote the replication of cells that might not have progressed into malignant tumors if not for the IGF-1 stimulation. IGF-1 stimulation is involved in a number of processes relevant to tumor growth: proliferation, survival, adhesion, migration, invasion, angiogenesis, and metastatic growth.[20]

Higher levels of IGF-1 have been associated with almost all cancers, though the largest amount of data available is for the most common cancers—of the breast, prostate, and colon. The European Prospective Investigation into Cancer and Nutrition (EPIC) found that elevated IGF-1 levels were associated with a 40 percent increased risk for breast cancer in postmenopausal women.[21] In the Nurses' Health Study, high IGF-1 levels were associated with a *doubling* in risk of breast cancer in premenopausal women.[22] Four meta-analyses have also associated elevated IGF-1 levels with breast cancer.[23] Elevated IGF-1 levels have also been associated with colorectal cancer, in research that demonstrated that IGF-1 promotes spread of colorectal cancer cells.[24] Finally, a 2009 meta-analysis of forty-two studies concluded that elevated circulating IGF-1 is associated with increased risk of prostate cancer.[25]

The combined effects of reduced IGF-1 and low levels of systemic inflammation have been proposed as a mechanism by which centenarians (those one hundred and older) are protected from cancer. Cellular inflammation is caused by excess free radicals and reactive oxygen species, as discussed earlier, and can be prevented by proper nutrition. So it is easy to see why the present dietary practices are so cancer-promoting. If you want to live to one hundred and thrive, you will require low levels of circulating IGF-1 and high levels of anti-inflammatory molecules. Genes signaling to enhance cells' DNA repair mechanisms to fight changes that could lead to cancer are supported by higher levels of anti-inflammatory molecules and plant micronutrients, and lower levels of IGF-1. The combined effect of a high-phytochemical diet resulting in reduced inflammation and oxidative stress, coupled with reduction in IGF-1, is the secret to maximizing longevity and cancer protection.[26]

Why Plant Protein Is Best

Amino acids are the individual building blocks of protein. Nine are called "essential," meaning that the body cannot make them from other amino acids. As noted earlier, consuming dietary proteins that are more "complete" in all essential amino acids—such as animal-source protein—causes larger increases in IGF-1 than does protein not as biologically complete and with more *non*essential amino acids. Generally, people with higher intake of animal products have much higher plasma IGF-1—that is, IGF-1 as measured in the blood—than those with lower intake.[27] In women, after adjusting for caloric intake, no association was found between fat or carbohydrate intake and IGF-1, but animal protein and milk drove up IGF-1 to risky levels. This suggests that a diet lower in animal protein is the most modifiable factor to maintain a lower and healthier level of IGF-1.[28]

Interestingly, saturated fat intake does not raise IGF-1 directly, but because it is associated with lower levels of IGF-binding proteins, it increases circulating free IGF-1 even further.[29] IGF-1 levels are also notably lower in vegans.[30]

Of all plant proteins, the essential amino acid distribution of soy is said to be the most "complete," meaning the closest to animal protein; soy has higher levels of many of the essential amino acids than other plant foods. While animal and soy proteins contain a greater content of essential amino acids, other plant proteins contain more than adequate amounts for human nutrition.[31] To discern the differences between the effects of soy and nonsoy plant protein, researchers broke down vegan women's protein intake further. They found that nonsoy plant protein was associated with lower IGF-1 levels, but soy protein was associated with higher IGF-1 levels.

It was noted by Dean Ornish's Prostate Cancer Lifestyle Trial that a low-fat vegan diet with supplemental soy protein did increase IGF-1, but it also increased the IGF-binding proteins; as a result, soy in moderate amounts did not have a significant effect on free IGF-1.[32] These results imply that soy protein, while it may raise IGF-1 levels, is still not as risky as animal protein. However, the more we concentrate these proteins and take them in an isolated form, the more potential they have to stimulate IGF-1 production. Dietary interventions using *isolated* soy protein have reported higher increases in IGF-1 than those using soybeans alone.[33] The bottom line: whole soybeans or minimally processed soy foods (such as tofu and tempeh) are acceptable; however, trying to build more muscle with *isolated* soy protein concentrates (such as powders) is not advisable.

High levels of IGF-1 are certainly detrimental to health, since they are strongly linked to cancers and also associated with all-cause mortality and cardiovascular mortality. Minimizing or avoiding animal protein and isolated soy protein should be the goal, to keep IGF-1 levels in a safe range. As for IGF-1 levels getting too *low*, you do not have to be concerned as long as you are eating a broad assortment of health-promoting plant foods.

The take-home message here is that animal protein—even egg whites and lean white meat—is not longevity-favorable and that our society's obsession with overconsuming protein is at the root of our epidemic of cancer. Super Immunity can only be achieved with a diet designed to be significantly lower in animal products than most of us consume today.

Reviewing Important Core Concepts

The key component to obtaining incredible health is to eat more vegetables, fruits, nuts and seeds, beans, and other nutrient-rich foods. As you eat larger amounts of these protective foods, you will meet your body's micronutrient needs and naturally reduce the amount of animal products and processed foods in your diet without gimmicks, calorie counting, or portion control. The foods highest in life-extending micronutrients and lowest in calories are green vegetables. As you know by now, they form the basis of my nutritarian diet. If you are overweight, the more greens you eat, and the less of everything else you eat, the thinner and healthier you will become. All humans are dependent on a sufficient amount of green vegetable–derived nutrients, and some of these nutrients should be consumed in their raw form for maximum benefit. This means that a large salad each day, with lettuce and other greens, tomatoes, and other raw vegetables, is important.

Eating high on the nutrient density line is important, but we also need enough nutritional variety to meet all the body's nutrient needs. To meet those needs in a manner that pushes your immune function to the max, you need to make sure your food choices cover all the bases that enable you to achieve Super Immunity. Here are five simple rules for a powerful immune system that you should commit to memory:

1. Eat a large salad every day.

2. Eat at least a half-cup serving of beans/legumes in soup, salad, or another dish once daily.

3. Eat at least three fresh fruits a day, especially berries, pomegranate seeds, cherries, plums, oranges.

4. Eat at least one ounce of raw nuts and seeds a day.

5. Eat at least one large (double-size) serving of green vegetables daily, either raw, steamed, or in soups or stews.

   Avoid these five deadliest foods:

1. Barbecued meat, processed meat, and commercial red meat

2. Fried foods

3. Full-fat dairy (cheese, ice cream, butter, whole milk) and trans fats (margarine)

4. Soft drinks, sugar, and artificial sweeteners

5. White-flour products

Now that you know what foods are *super* foods and what you should be eating for Super Immunity, the question is how much processed food, french fries, pizza, burgers, and fried rice you can eat and still be protected. And if you love meat, I bet you're wondering how much animal product you can eat and still stay healthy.

The answer? I don't know for sure, and nobody does—but my review of the world's scientific literature over the last twenty years suggests that the combination of processed foods and animal products should comprise less than 10 percent of your total caloric intake; go beyond that and you start to pay a significant price in health issues. In general, try to eat not more than one or two foods a day that are not health-supporting.

NUTRIENT DENSITY SCORES OF THE TOP 25 SUPER FOODS

To make it easy for you to achieve Super Immunity, I've listed my Top 25 Super Foods below. These foods are associated with protection against cancer and promotion of a long, healthy life. Include as many of these foods in your diet as you possibly can. *You are what you eat. To be your best, you must eat the best!*

Collard, mustard, turnip greens 1000

Kale 1000

Watercress 1000

Swiss chard 895

Bok choy 865

Cabbage (all varieties) 434–715

Spinach 707

Arugula 604

Lettuce (Boston, romaine, red and green leaf) 367–585

Brussels sprouts 490

Carrots 458

Broccoli 340

Cauliflower 315

Bell peppers, red and green 207–265

Mushrooms 238

Asparagus 205

Tomatoes 185

Berries (all varieties) 132–182

Pomegranates 119

Grapes 119

Cantaloupe 118

Onions 109

Seeds: flax, sunflower, sesame, hemp, chia (avg) 39–103

Beans (all varieties) 43–98

Nuts (all varieties) 26–60

If you are a female eating between 1,400 and 1,800 calories a day, only 150 calories a day should come from animal products and refined carbohydrates (such as you'd find in a cookie or white pasta). The remainder of the food should come from natural plant foods such as green vegetables, beans, seeds, and nuts. If you are a male and eating between 1,800 and 2,400 calories a day, no more than 200 calories should be from these foods.

This means that if you're using a few tablespoons of oil, you've used up your allotment of low-nutrient calories. So if you're having an animal protein for dinner, don't have the oil. Or if you're eating a bagel, don't have the animal protein.

Whole-grain bread, whole-grain pasta, and whole-grain cereal would not have to be considered in this limit, of course. Only products made of white flour or processed grains would fall in the processed food category.

Keep in mind that 150 and 200 calories are the daily low-nutrient limits for most women and men. The following list shows some examples of foods and indicates how much of each food it takes to wipe out your daily calorie allotment:

	150 CALORIES	200 CALORIES
Olive oil	1.25 tablespoons	1.75 tablespoons
Chicken breast	3.2 ounces	4.3 ounces
Pizza	0.5 slice	0.75 slice
French fries	15 fries	20 fries
Bagel	0.8 bagel	1.1 bagel
White pasta	0.7 cup	0.9 cup
Scrambled eggs	1.5 eggs	2 eggs
Milk (1 percent)	12 ounces	15 ounces
Skim milk	14 ounces	19 ounces
Oatmeal cookie	2 cookies	2.5 cookies
Salmon	3.8 ounces	5.1 ounces
Tilapia	4.2 ounces	5.5 ounces
Lean beef (broiled)	2.1 ounces	2.8 ounces
Cheddar cheese	1.3 ounces	1.7 ounces

When it comes to the animal products or the processed foods you choose to eat, make sure you're making the best choices given what's available. Fast-food hamburgers made from factory-bred cows are just too dangerous a food to consume on a regular or even limited basis.

So I recommend choosing eggs, grass-fed meats, clean wild fish, and naturally raised, hormone-free poultry. Likewise, when it comes to sweets, homemade is always better, with dried or fresh fruit as the sweetening agent, not conventional sweeteners. Speaking of homemade, why not have a delicious cookie, cake, or ice cream from choices supplied in the recipe section that concludes this book?

Over time most nutritarians (including me) come to *enjoy* the healthier options more than the conventional fast, junk, or overly processed foods. Once you start eating for health, these other options will become less and less appealing, and before too long any cravings or desires will simply disappear.

More good news is that my years of experience in the nutrition field have led to wonderful relationships with top chefs the world over. And what I can report is that from the top chefs down, the quality and super-healthy nature of what's available is beginning to change. "Gourmet" no longer means a hunk of meat with a large side of creamy potatoes. We now have some of the best chefs in the world making the healthiest foods. We can have an immune-supporting, cancer-protective diet—and make it great-tasting as well.

A survey of thousands of nutritarians adopting this diet-style for health and longevity found that after an adjustment period of a few months, the vast majority eventually enjoyed the new foods and recipes as much as or more than their old diets.[34] What may seem radical at the moment will soon become delicious and life-changing.

CHAPTER SIX

Making the Right Choices

E very day we have hundreds of choices to make about what we put into our bodies. Some of these choices can be difficult to navigate without the facts. There is a great deal of misinformation floating around, and time and again I have seen individuals make important health decisions based on faulty information. Through my practice working with patients, I have answered and continue to answer tens of thousands of specific questions about these very choices.

In the pages that follow I have carefully selected the most important and practical information we need to know—everything from quantities of animal protein and salt, to sources for omega-3s, to dos and don'ts of vitamin supplements. I provide specific recommendations that answer some of the most debated questions in the health field, supported by the latest scientific data available.

It is important to remember that changing the way you eat may not happen overnight. However, thousands of people have already made this change and found that it was easier and more delicious than they expected. As your health improves with superior nutrition, your taste buds also get stronger and you learn to love what you are eating. It takes time to create new food preferences, but the wait will be worth it—and my recipes make it delicious too.

Throughout the book, I have offered guidelines for you on your path to Super Immunity. Because of the research done in the field of nutritional science, we have at our disposal all the facts we need. We know the foods that can lead to a long, healthy life, just as we know the foods and choices that can lead to deteriorating health. The effort you expend to improve your health pays you back one hundredfold. Your good health forms the basis of your success and happiness in life.

Choosing the right foods has the power to save your life. Let's start this journey together today.

Vegan vs. Near-Vegan

A question commonly asked of me is if a vegan diet, one totally free of animal products, is better or more health-promoting than a diet that includes a small amount of animal products.

The unbiased, scientific answer is that nobody knows for sure. Even though vegans have lower heart attack rates and generally lower cancer rates than the conventional population, those same benefits are documented in people who follow healthy diets that include the occasional consumption of animal products. This includes, for example, near-vegetarians who eat meat or fish about once a week.[1] A review of five mortality studies on this issue showed that those who ate fish occasionally had statistics that were just as impressive as those of the vegans. The longest-lived societies in recorded history—such as the Hunzas in central Asia, the Abkhazians in southern Russia, the Vilcabambans in the Andes of South America, and the Okinawans in Japan—all ate very little animal products but were not completely vegan.[2] As we drift considerably up from the occasional use of animal products, to include animal products in significant amounts, we see evidence that more heart disease and most cancers become more prevalent.[3] Clearly, it is the combination of more fruits and vegetables in conjunction with a reduction in animal products that offers us the greatest opportunity for longevity.[4]

In the United States, the most significant research clarifying this issue studied Seventh-Day Adventists, a religious group useful to study for this purpose because nearly all members avoid tobacco and alcohol and follow a generally health-promoting lifestyle. About half of them are vegetarian, while the other half consume modest amounts of meat. The Adventists' lifestyle allowed scientists to separate the effects of not eating meat from other health-promoting practices. The researchers even tracked those who ate animal products just once a week—the near-vegetarians, as they called them. This twelve-year study, published in the 2001 *Archives of Internal Medicine,* found that Seventh-Day Adventists in the United States were the longest-lived population ever formally studied. The strict vegetarian (vegan) females had the longest average lifespan, 85.7 years (over six years longer than that of the average female Californian), and the males 83.3 years (nine and a half years longer than that of the average male Californian). The longest-lived were those vegetarians who ate nuts and seeds regularly; the nut-eating vegans lived slightly longer than the near-vegetarians. The effect of eating nuts and seeds regularly was more significantly linked to enhanced lifespan than was the strictness of the vegan diet. This means that those on a near-vegan diet, with the regular consumption of nuts and seeds, had better longevity statistics than the strict vegans who did not eat nuts and seeds. Overall, studies on longevity show significant reductions in cancer risk among those who avoided meat.[5]

The contemporary diet in America and many other countries includes over 25 percent of calories from animal products. As I hope the preceding chapter made clear, after my lifetime of study of this issue, carefully evaluating all the science and supporting evidence, it is obvious that there should no longer be any controversy: the preponderance of evidence is overwhelming and conclusive that to maximize longevity we need to reduce consumption of animal products and instead eat more plant products. A legitimate question for further research is whether my estimate of the 10 percent of calories from animal products as an upper limit is sufficiently restrictive to maximize lifespan if the diet is otherwise excellent.

The problem is that there are very few who can study this issue without their predetermined bias affecting their judgment. In modern times, nutrition has become like politics, with camps of various persuasions believing in the righteousness of their approach. Each camp has a mission, agenda, and ego to protect. Some high-protein, low-carbohydrate dietary gurus actually promote more than double the amount of animal products already consumed, under the misconception that raising intake of animal protein will result in satisfactory weight-loss outcomes and better health. Whether some people can lose some weight on such a plan or not is almost irrelevant, if the price they pay is a much earlier death. You could smoke cigarettes to lose weight too!

On the other hand, the vegan diet movement also frequently uses the available science in a selective way, proposing and interpreting studies in a way that supports a diet completely free of animal products. That is not to say there aren't lots of ethical and environmental arguments that justify a vegan diet and its value to mankind. But I am a nutritional scientist, researcher, and physician, and my job is to make sure my advice is not tempered by ancillary motivations and personal views, but sticks to the science of nutrition and health, my expertise. A true scientist tests a theory without a predetermined agenda and collects not just the facts favorable to his or her position, but *all* the facts.

A totally vegan diet is deficient in B_{12}, and may result in suboptimal levels of EPA and DHA (eicosapentaenoic acid and docosahexaenoic acid), those long-chain beneficial fats commonly found in wild salmon and sardines. If we were living in ancient times, with no potential to supplement a vegan diet with vitamin B_{12}, then it would be an inappropriate option. But today it is easy to supplement judiciously, to ensure that no potential deficiencies occur; and we can even do blood work to ascertain if the levels are optimal. That means a vegan diet becomes not just a legitimate option, but maybe even the healthiest option of all dietary patterns.

The inclusion of fish for beneficial fatty acids may be of some benefit to a subset of vegans, who do not naturally make ideal amounts of the long-chain omega-3 fats found in fish. This is more of a concern for those who are aging, as the ability to self-manufacture sufficient long-chain fats decreases in the elderly; and in my experience, a deficiency in this area is more prevalent in males. But even this can be checked with a blood test and supplemented by vegan forms of EPA and DHA to assure ideal levels, without the need to eat fish.

Iodine and zinc are other nutrients of concern in the vegan diet, though the majority of individuals on vegan diets are not deficient; again, blood tests can be utilized to confirm adequacy. Furthermore, adding a small amount of iodine to the diet is easily accomplished with a pinch of kelp a few times each week, or with an appropriate supplement to supply extra zinc, iodine, B_{12}, and vitamin D. Vitamin D, the sunshine vitamin, is also not found in adequate amounts in food and should be supplemented appropriately in those not exposed to sufficient sunshine.

Given the information presented in the preceding chapters, you should understand the benefits of certain plants to enhance immune function and the need to increase their consumption as a percentage of total calories. It is necessary to restrict both processed foods and animal products to have room in the caloric pie to take in adequate amounts of foods rich in cancer-protective nutrients. This is how you get the additional benefit that reduces the biological and hormonal effects of animal foods to promote heart disease and cancer. Furthermore, if you accept the science and logic that a diet rich in micronutrients per calorie potentiates longevity, that automatically makes restriction of animal products a necessity. Some people may choose to eat more animal products than I recommend, and many will defend their food preferences to their death. But we should all recognize that this is not a well-informed choice—and not one made on health issues alone, but influenced by factors such as personal preference.

The Transition to Fewer Animal Products

Many people claim to need animal products to feel good and perform well. In my experience, this assertion generally comes from individuals who felt worse during the first couple of weeks after a change to a lower-animal-source diet. Instead of being patient, they simply returned to their old way of eating—genuinely feeling better for it—and now insist that they *need* meat to thrive.

A diet heavily burdened with animal products places a huge stress on the detoxification systems of the body. As with stopping caffeine and cigarettes, many people observe withdrawal symptoms for a short period, usually including fatigue, weakness, headaches, or loose stools. In 95 percent of such cases, these symptoms resolve within two weeks. It is more common that the temporary adjustment period, during which you might feel mild symptoms as your body withdraws from your prior toxic habits, lasts less than a week.

Unfortunately, many people mistakenly assume these symptoms to be due to some lack in the new diet and go back to eating a poor diet again. Sometimes they have been convinced that they feel bad because they aren't eating enough protein, especially since when they return to their old diet they feel better again. People often confuse *feeling* well with *getting* well, not realizing that sometimes you have to temporarily feel a little worse to really get well.

Don't buy the fallacy that you need more protein. The dietary program recommended here and in my other books offers sufficient protein—and protein deficiency does not cause long-term fatigue. Even my vegan menus supply about 50 grams of protein per 1,000 calories, a whopping amount.

One of the most common symptoms that occurs when someone lowers the amount of animal protein and eliminates sweets from the diet is *temporary* fatigue. This is just part of the normal detoxification process that most people have to get through. Again, this process most often results in mild symptoms that last less than five days.

Reducing salt intake suddenly can also cause fatigue from a lowering of blood pressure, which occurs from a temporary dip of sodium in the bloodstream as the kidneys adjust. It could take a few weeks for the kidneys, accustomed to dumping a huge sodium load (from a high-salt diet), to recognize that they need to stop removing so much sodium from the system. This initial miscalculation contributes to the fatigue experienced the first week after a major change in one's diet.

Other symptoms, such as increased gas and loose stools, are also occasionally observed when people switch to a diet containing abundant fiber—and *different* fibers, ones that the digestive tract has never encountered before. Over many years, the body has adjusted its secretions and peristaltic waves (intestinal contractions as food moves through) to a low-fiber diet. These symptoms also improve with time. Chewing especially well, sometimes even blending salads, helps in this period of transition. Some people must use beans only in small amounts initially, increasing them gradually over a period of weeks to train the digestive track to handle and digest these new fibers.

There are some individuals with increased dietary requirements for protein who have to plan their plant-based, nutritarian diet to include more protein-rich foods. Sunflower seeds, hemp seeds, Mediterranean pine nuts, and soybeans are all options to meet this higher requirement with plant sources of protein. Certain people have increased fat requirements too, and if they tried out a vegetarian diet in the past, it may not have been rich enough in certain essential fats for them. This can occur in those eating a plant-based diet that includes lots of low-fat wheat and grain products. Adding ground flax seeds and walnuts to the diet to supply additional omega-3 fats is helpful.

Some people, especially thin individuals, require more calories and more fat to sustain their weight. This is usually resolved by including raw nuts, raw nut butters, avocados, and other healthy foods that are nutrient-rich *and* high in fat and calories. Even these naturally thin individuals will significantly improve their health and lower their risk of degenerative diseases if they reduce their dependency on animal foods and instead consume more plant-derived fats, such as those in nuts.

Last, there is the rare individual who needs more concentrated sources of protein and fat in his diet because of digestive impairment, Crohn's disease, short bowel syndrome, or other unique medical conditions. I have also encountered patients on rare occasions who require more protein because of a particular lack: these individuals, because of their genetics, do not manufacture ideal amounts of one or more of the nonessential amino acids, usually the amino acid taurine. On these rare occasions, an amino acid supplement or more animal product is needed to slow transit time in the gut, and to aid absorption and concentration of amino acids at each meal. This problem can also be the result of some digestive impairment or difficulty with absorption. However, it would be exceedingly rare that an individual who combined high-protein seeds with a taurine supplement and the small amount of animal products I advise would have to eat a diet with a higher amount of animal products to thrive. These rare individuals should still follow my general recommendations for excellent health, and can accommodate their individual needs by keeping animal protein down to comparatively low levels.

Exercise's Effect on Immunity and Lifespan

People who exercise regularly have fewer and milder colds—at least that's what we tend to hear. Exercise enthusiasts always brag that they're sick less than sedentary people.

Before this was well studied, nobody really knew how true it was. In one particular study, the researchers collected data on 1,002 men and women from ages eighteen to eighty-five. Over twelve weeks in the autumn and winter of 2008, the researchers tracked the number of upper-respiratory-tract infections the participants suffered. The study accounted for a variety of factors, including age, body mass index, and education. Participants were also quizzed about their lifestyle, dietary patterns, and stressful events, all of which can affect the immune system. In addition, all the participants reported how much and what kinds of aerobic exercise they did weekly, and rated their fitness levels using a ten-point system.

The researchers found that the frequency of colds among people who exercised five or more days a week was up to 46 percent less than that of people who were largely sedentary—that is, who exercised only one day or less per week. These results are stunning—half the number of viral infections for those who were exercising regularly! Furthermore, when these individuals *did* come down with an illness, it was not as severe an illness, and the number of days of being ill was a whopping 41 percent less.[6]

Exercise not only helps your immune system fight off simple bacterial and viral infections; it also decreases your chances of developing heart disease, osteoporosis, and cancer. The key to the longevity-promoting effects of exercise is maintaining a high degree of exercise tolerance and fitness.

When middle-aged men were followed for twenty-six years, researchers found that those who exercised vigorously lived the longest.[7] It truly is survival of the fittest! The same thing is true regarding heart disease prevention.[8] In other words, it is not sufficient just to take walks; adding on more exerting exercise, where the heart rate is elevated, and sustaining that elevation for at least five minutes has additional benefits.

I advise you to exercise vigorously, with jogging, jumping in place, and other heart-rate-elevating exercises or activities. Keep your leg muscles and the central muscles in the abdomen and back strong. To achieve maximum benefit, exercise at least three days per week.

That does *not* mean that being involved in competitive triathlons or marathons is lifespan-enhancing. *Extreme* exercise is a major stress on the body and produces excessive free radicals. In most cases, the benefits that vigorous exercise gives us, including the increased functional efficiency in almost all the body's cells, more than compensates for the added physical stress. However, with *extreme* degrees of vigorous exercise, such as extended-length events of competitive running, biking, or cross-country skiing, the stress on the body can exceed the benefits.

What You Need to Know About Vitamins and Nutritional Supplements

First of all, I recommend for most individuals a high-quality multivitamin/multimineral capsule to assure favorable levels of vitamin D, B_{12}, zinc, and iodine. Very few of us eat perfectly, and it makes sense to be sure that you ingest adequate amounts of these important substances, especially those nutrients whose levels may be less than ideal even with an excellent diet.

Making sure we have enough iodine is vital, especially because our diet change will limit the amount of salt we ingest. Most grocery store salt has been iodinated, making it the primary source of iodine in most people's diets. Zinc, as discussed earlier, is an essential mineral that can be difficult to ingest in adequate amounts through a healthy diet. For example, zinc does not often reach ideal levels on a vegan or near-vegan diet. Therefore, the right multivitamin can assure adequate iodine and zinc intake to keep our immune systems functioning at an optimal level. However, as you will see, we have to be careful about the other components of the multivitamin.

A Word of Caution

I have carefully reviewed the studies on every typical multivitamin/multimineral ingredient, and there is clearly a significant risk from supplementing certain nutrients on a regular basis, especially in the dosages found in high-potency vitamin supplements. So even though multivitamins may contain beneficial nutrients, they also contain ingredients that are harmful and may significantly increase one's risk of cancer.

Vitamin and mineral use generally follows a biphasic dose response curve. This means that too little is a problem, a certain middle range is likely ideal, and too much can cause a problem as well. This curve can be clearly observed if we look at the data on vitamin E. Whereas eating foods rich in vitamin E and the various vitamin E fragments is clearly beneficial, taking a *large* dose, such as 200–400 international units (or IU, a standard measure of vitamin potency)—an amount unobtainable from even the richest vitamin E–containing foods—has negative effects.[9]

Here's what we need to look out for. The riskiest nutrients in a supplement are vitamin A (retinyl acetate or retinyl palmitate) and folic acid. These two nutrients account for the negative aspects of most multivitamins and detract from the overall benefits of taking a typical multi. The strong negative effects of supplemental vitamin A and folic acid may account for why studies on multivitamins are so inconclusive, with some studies showing benefits and others showing none. Overall, there is insufficient evidence to conclude that a multivitamin, as currently constituted, plays a significant role in extending lifespan or reducing the incidence of cancer. However, since science has shown that the negative effects come from only a limited number of supplemental ingredients (discussed below), with the strongest negative effects from folic acid and vitamin A, a study conducted on a properly designed multivitamin, without those ingredients, would probably reveal health benefits.

This potential for a multi, without vitamin A and folic acid, to offer health or lifespan benefits is supported by the evidence that the general use of a multivitamin extends the length of cellular telomeres, which protect chromosomes and help ensure normal DNA replication. Subjects taking a multi were found to have over 5 percent longer telomeres compared to those who did not take a multi on a regular basis.

Telemeres shorten with aging, and shorter telomeres are associated with shorter lifespan.[10]

Let's look at some of the potentially troublesome elements of a multivitamin/multimineral in more detail.

Beta-Carotene

Ingesting vitamin A or beta-carotene in isolation—from supplements, instead of from food—may interfere with the absorption of other crucially important carotenoids, such as lutein and lycopene, thus potentially increasing cancer risk.[11] Beta-carotene once was regarded as a safe and beneficial antioxidant and even recommended as an anticancer vitamin, but it has recently been shown to increase the risk of certain cancers when administered as a supplement rather than ingested from food. Scientists now suspect that problems may result when beta-carotene is ingested without other carotenoids that would have been present had it been ingested from real food. Beta-carotene is only one of about five hundred carotenoids that exist. Beta-carotene supplements are poor substitutes for the broad assortment of carotenoid compounds found in plants.

Years ago scientists noted that populations with high levels of beta-carotene in their bloodstream had exceedingly low rates of cancer. Now we understand that the reason these people were protected against cancer was the hundreds of *other* carotenoids and phytochemicals in the fruits and vegetables they were consuming. Beta-carotene served as a flag or marker for those populations with a high fruit and vegetable intake. Unfortunately, many people confused the flag for the ship.

In Finnish trials, people using beta-carotene supplements not only failed to prevent lung cancer; there was actually an increase in cancer in those who took the supplement.[12] This study was halted when the researchers (physicians) discovered that the death rate from lung cancer was 28 percent higher among participants who had taken the high amounts of beta-carotene and vitamin A. Furthermore, the death rate from heart disease was 17 percent higher in those who had taken the supplements compared to those given a placebo.

Vitamin A

Since beta-carotene gets converted into vitamin A by your body, there is no reason why a person eating a reasonably healthy diet would require any extra vitamin A. The ingestion of extra vitamin A is even riskier than the ingestion of supplemental beta-carotene. In humans, excess vitamin A is potentially a problem, even in ranges not normally considered toxic. A Cochrane review of sixty-eight randomized trials of vitamin A supplementation (with a mean dose of 20,000 IU) showed an average of 16 percent increase mortality risk (mean three years).[13] This means that excess vitamin A is a risk for cancer, and that risk is significant.

There is also a major concern that supplemental vitamin A induces calcium loss in the urine, contributing to osteoporosis. Even though too much vitamin A is known to be toxic to the liver, the most common effect of toxic doses of vitamin A in animals is spontaneous fracture. Apparently, excess vitamin A is potentially a problem for human bones too[14]—one study showed a doubling of the hip fracture rate comparing vitamin A intake in the .5 milligram range to the 1.5 milligram range.[15] This is the 1,500 IU to 4,500 IU range, the typical amount found in most vitamin supplements. Vitamin A has also been linked to birth defects.

Folic Acid

First, please note that *folate* is not the same thing as *folic acid*, though many people use these terms interchangeably. Folate is a member of the B vitamin family and is found naturally in plant foods, especially green vegetables. It is involved with DNA methylation, which essentially turns genes on and off. This critical role makes folate important in fetal development and nerve tissue health as well as cancer initiation and progression.

Due to folate's important role in DNA processing and human development, women are told to take folic acid in a prenatal supplement during pregnancy to prevent neural-tube birth defects. The problem is that folic acid is not the same as the folate found in real food. Folic acid is not found in natural foods at all; it is the synthetic form of folate that is used as an ingredient in vitamin supplements. Folic acid is also added to most enriched, refined grain products like bread, rice, and pasta in the United States and Canada, in an attempt to replace the nutrients lost during the processing of whole grains.

Because folic acid is added to so many refined grain products, it is very easy for a typical diet combined with a multivitamin to end up with high levels of folic acid. Too much folate obtained naturally from food is not a concern; only the synthetic form is suspect. Scientists do not yet know the implications of circulating synthetic folic acid, but more and more evidence suggests that supplementing with folic acid increases the occurrence of certain cancers.

Folate is abundant in all green vegetables. We do *not* need synthetic folic acid supplements to meet our daily folate requirements. Listed below are a few examples of folate-rich foods. (As a reference point, the U.S. RDI for folate is 400 micrograms.)

MICROGRAMS OF FOLATE IN FOLATE-RICH FOODS

Asparagus (1.5 cup cooked)	402
Edamame (1 cup cooked)	358
Lentils (1 cup cooked)	358
Broccoli (2 cups cooked)	337
Chickpeas (1 cup cooked)	282
Adzuki beans (1 cup cooked)	278
Romaine lettuce (3 cups raw)	192
Brussels sprouts (2 cups cooked)	187
Spinach (3 cups raw)	175

Recent studies have demonstrated significant concerns about folic acid:

- Women who took extra folic acid during pregnancy were followed by researchers for thirty years, and they were found to be twice as likely to die from breast cancer as women who had no folic acid supplementation.[16]

- Another study following women for ten years concluded that those who took multivitamins containing folic acid increased their breast cancer risk by 20 to 30 percent.[17]

- Folic acid supplementation by pregnant women has been associated with a higher incidence (in their offspring) of childhood asthma, infant respiratory tract infections, and cardiac birth defects.[18]

- Men who took folic acid supplements for more than three years had a 35 percent increase in colorectal cancer risk, with increasing precancerous colorectal adenomas, according to a meta-analysis of several randomized controlled trials.[19]

- In a ten-year study, folic acid supplementation was associated with more than double the risk of prostate cancer compared to placebos.[20]

- In two trials comparing folic acid supplements to placebos, overall cancer incidence and all-cause mortality were increased in the folic acid group over the nine-year study period.[21]

- Recently, in Norway, where they do not fortify their flour with folic acid, researchers conducted a six-year study on the homocysteine-lowering effects of B vitamins for patients with heart disease. Unexpectedly, they found that those whose supplements contained folic acid were 43 percent more likely to die from cancer.[22]

In contrast, higher levels of *food-derived* folate are associated with less breast and prostate cancer.[23] Furthermore, when you get your folate from produce, you get thousands of other beneficial cancer-fighting nutrients in the process.

As I have already stated, health authorities have emphasized the critical importance of taking folic acid supplements during pregnancy to prevent birth defects of the spinal cord. Almost all women are aware of these recommendations, and the matter is emphasized by all physicians. Is this the right approach? I think it is clear now that it was and is a big mistake. Instead, health authorities should be emphasizing the need for childbearing women to eat sufficient greens and beans each day.

Our present system, where women rely on a pill and not on real foods, leads to a plethora of serious health problems in children— among them, the conditions mentioned in the research list above: childhood asthma, infant respiratory tract infections, and cardiac birth defects. On the other hand, the children of women who consumed more *food* folate during pregnancy were less likely to develop attention deficit hyperactivity disorder (ADHD).[24] Even more startling is the reduction of childhood cancers seen in the children of women who consumed folate-containing green foods during pregnancy and did not take folic acid supplements.[25]

My contention is that the reliance on folic acid during pregnancy, instead of educating women about the importance of consuming natural food for their folate needs, is permitting an epidemic of childhood leukemia, which could have been easily prevented. Women should also be aware that consuming processed meats during pregnancy (or even in the year prior to conception) increases the risk of their child having cancer, including leukemia and brain tumors.[26]

Getting enough *folate* from natural foods can keep cancers from starting, by repairing errors in DNA, but *folic acid* appears to feed tumor development and promote carcinogenesis. In light of this research, I do not include folic acid in my multivitamin or prenatal vitamin. I do not recommend that pregnant women take a prenatal that contains folic acid. I do recommend a blood test for folate sufficiency before even contemplating pregnancy, and I do recommend a high-folate diet rich in green vegetables. A diet that includes the regular consumption of green vegetables is the safest way to protect your offspring and achieve protection from cancer, heart disease, and all-cause mortality.

Copper and Iron

Recent studies have shown that excess copper could be associated with reduced immune function and lower antioxidant status.[27] Recently published research also indicates that high copper intake combined with a diet high in saturated and trans fats could lead to an accelerated rate of mental decline in older adults.[28] Caution here is warranted, and it is prudent not to supplement with copper.

Iron should also not be supplemented in males or postmenopausal women who no longer bleed regularly. Iron is an oxidant and can contribute to infection and even increase heart attack risk.[29] It should be taken as a supplement only when a deficiency or enhanced need exists.

Beyond these above-discussed elements, there is no evidence that other nutrients in the RDI dose ranges found in ordinary multivitamin/multimineral preparations are harmful. However a crucial point needs to be made: *supplements are not substitutes for a healthy diet.* To the extent that they offer some people the confidence to eat less wholesome vegetation, they are hurtful, not helpful.

The Role of Probiotics and Fermented Foods

As we saw in an earlier chapter, approximately one-third of the dry weight of our stool is bacteria. Shortly after birth, promoted by bacterial growth factors in human breast milk, the digestive tract gradually gets colonized with about thirty to fifty different species of beneficial bacteria. These bacteria serve a host of useful functions, including repressing the growth of harmful organisms, training the immune system to respond to only pathogenic bacteria, detoxifying and removing cancer-causing toxins, and producing immune system–supporting nutrients. The natural, native bacterial flora of humans also protect against allergies and immune disorders by decreasing absorption of incompletely digested proteins.

The term "probiotics" is used both for the beneficial bacteria that are native to our intestinal tract and for supplemental live bacterial organisms that are thought to be beneficial when ingested. However, the (limited) bacteria in supplemental probiotics and fermented foods are not the same as the indigenous bacterial flora that live in the gut. Supplemental probiotics serve a beneficial role—but mostly when the normal native bacteria have been harmed or removed with antibiotic use or perverted with a diet of sweets and processed foods.

There is no published evidence that probiotic supplements are able to effectively replace all the functions of the body's natural flora when these have been killed off. Probiotics are useful after taking antibiotics, as noted; but it can still take months to reestablish the normal type and amount of gut flora. Healthy foods promote healthy bacteria to live in the gut; unhealthy foods promote unhealthy bacteria and yeast forms. However, unless a healthy diet, rich in various fibers, is continually maintained, the probiotic bacterial levels achieved by supplements drop within days when supplementation ceases. So what we eat is still the most important factor in maintaining our intestinal flora.

"Good" bacteria feast on fiber and resistant starch, while "bad" bacteria and yeast feast on refined sugar and animal fat. There is no substitute for a healthy diet; and if you are eating health-promoting foods and avoiding junk foods and antibiotics, it is not necessary for you to take probiotics or fermented foods. Your body will grow the right kind of bacteria automatically.

One of the complications of antibiotic therapy is secondary infection—a huge problem in hospitals. Until recently there hasn't been a good understanding of how and why this occurs. Now researchers have identified the way that normal gut flora keep the immune system "primed" to recognize the cell walls of bacteria so that the slightest change from a normal to a pathogenic bacterium will stimulate an immediate attack.[30] Antibiotics shut this recognition ability down, leaving the body without one of its defense systems. Probiotics can help turn this safeguard back on again.

If you are taking antibiotics more than once per year, then of course the continual use of probiotics is recommended, as it could take a year or more to reestablish normal bacterial protection each time. Otherwise, probiotics should be used for at least three months after each use of antibiotics. Fortunately, most healthy people eating a healthy diet should never need an antibiotic—not once in their life—because dangerous bacterial infections are exceedingly rare in people with excellent immunity.

Probiotic supplements may be indicated and helpful for certain other conditions as well, such as irritable bowel syndrome, autoimmune diseases, allergies, headaches, and excessive yeast in the gut. They are also helpful for those who are not eating properly for good health.

More than a dozen studies on the effectiveness of probiotics in preventing viral infections such as colds and flu have been conducted, with mixed results. Most studies have shown some decrease in the severity and number of illness days in participants randomly assigned to treatment groups.[31] The inconsistency of the evidence demonstrates that probiotics are more useful for unhealthy people eating unhealthfully, and less helpful for those eating healthfully and in good general health.

A healthy diet with plenty of raw vegetables, mushrooms, and beans, in the absence of antibiotics, will provide enough of the favorable bacteria in your gut to you keep you healthy and functioning at your highest levels. It is not necessary to eat fermented foods such as yogurt and kefir to have beneficial bacteria in the digestive tract. However, the more a person consumes sweets and processed foods and utilizes antibiotics, the more likely it is that he or she will require ongoing supplementation with probiotics.

Probiotics are well tolerated in adults, children, pregnant women, and even premature infants. However, they should be avoided in severely immune-compromised patients with HIV or advanced cancer or people undergoing chemotherapy.

Salt Intake

Table salt consists of sodium chloride. It supplies us with sodium, an important mineral that is essential for proper functioning of the human body. However, the American diet contains dangerously high amounts of sodium, almost 80 percent of which comes from processed and restaurant foods. The human diet, for millions of years, did not contain *any* added salt—only the sodium present in natural foods, which adds up to about 600–800 milligrams per day. The dietary intake of sodium in the United States today is about 3,500 milligrams per day.

Excess dietary salt is most notorious for increasing blood pressure. Populations in pockets of the world that do not salt their food do not have elderly citizens with high blood pressure (also known as hypertension). Americans have a 90 percent lifetime probability of developing high blood pressure. So even if your blood pressure is normal now, if you continue to eat the typical American diet, you will be at risk.

Elevated blood pressure accounts for 62 percent of strokes and 49 percent of coronary heart disease.[32] Notably, the risk for heart attack and stroke begins climbing with systolic pressures (the first number in the blood pressure reading) above 115—considered "normal" by most standards. Even if you eat an otherwise healthy diet, and your arteries are free of plaque, hypertension late in life damages the delicate blood vessels of the brain, increasing the risk of hemorrhagic stroke.

The American Heart Association, recognizing the significant risks of high blood pressure, has recently dropped their recommended maximum daily sodium intake from 2,300 milligrams to 1,500 milligrams.

Salt has additional dangerous effects that are not related to blood pressure. In the 1990s, it was found that the relationship between salt intake and stroke mortality was stronger than the relationship between blood pressure and stroke mortality; this result suggests that salt may have deleterious effects on the cardiovascular system that are not related to blood pressure.[33] Likewise, high blood pressure causes kidney disease, but dietary sodium has damaging effects on the kidneys beyond the indirect effects of high blood pressure.[34]

Further research has determined that long-term excess dietary sodium promotes excessive cell growth, leading to thickening of the vessel walls and altered production of structural proteins, leading to stiff blood vessels. In another study, higher sodium intake was associated with greater carotid artery wall thickness, an accurate predictor of future heart attacks and strokes—even in people without high blood pressure.[35]

High salt intake is also a risk factor for osteoporosis, because excess dietary sodium promotes urinary calcium loss, leading to calcium loss from bones (and therefore decreased bone density). Daily sodium intakes characteristic of Americans have been associated with increased bone loss at the hip, and sodium restriction reduces markers of bone breakdown. Even in the presence of a high-calcium diet, high salt intake results in net calcium loss from bone.[36]

Although postmenopausal women are most vulnerable to these calcium losses, high salt intake in young girls may prevent the attainment of peak bone mass during puberty, putting these girls at risk for osteoporosis later in life.

Salt is also the strongest factor relating to stomach cancer. Sodium intake statistics from twenty-four countries have been significantly correlated to stomach cancer mortality rates. Additional studies have found positive correlations between salt consumption and gastric cancer incidence.[37] A high-salt diet also increases growth of the ulcer-promoting bacteria (*H. pylori*) in the stomach, which is a risk factor for gastric cancer.[38] Alarmingly, high sodium intake also correlates with death from all causes.[39]

Reducing dietary salt is not only important for those who already have elevated blood pressure; limiting added salt is essential for *all* of us to remain in good health. Since natural foods supply us with 600–800 milligrams of sodium a day, it is wise to limit any additional sodium, over and above what is in natural food, to just a few hundred milligrams. I recommend no more than 1,000 milligrams total of sodium per day. That means not more than 200–400 milligrams over and above what is found in your natural foods.

It is also important to note that expensive and exotic sea salts are still salt. *All* salt originates from the sea—and so-called sea salts are still over 98 percent sodium chloride, contributing the same amount of sodium per teaspoon as regular salt. Sea salts may contain small amounts of trace minerals, but the amounts are insignificant compared to those in natural plant foods, and the excess sodium doesn't magically become less harmful due to those minerals. A high-nutrient, vegetable-based diet with little or no added salt is ideal.

Salt also deadens the taste buds. This means that if you avoid highly salted and processed foods, you will regain your ability to detect and enjoy the subtle flavors in natural foods and actually experience heightened pleasure from natural, unsalted foods.

Since most salt comes from processed foods, avoiding added sodium isn't difficult. Resist adding salt to foods, and purchase salt-free canned goods and soups. If you must salt your food, do so only after it is on the table and you are ready to eat it—it will taste saltier if the salt is right on the surface. Condiments such as ketchup, mustard, soy sauce, teriyaki sauce, and relish are all high in sodium. Use garlic, onion, fresh or dried herbs, spices, lemon or lime juice, or vinegar to flavor food. Experiment to find salt-free seasonings that you enjoy.

The Coffee Question

I am often questioned about the health effects of coffee: Can a healthy diet include coffee? Is coffee actually *good* for people?

The good news first. Mysterious protective effects of coffee against diabetes have been reported. A 2010 meta-analysis analyzing data from eighteen studies reported that each additional cup of coffee consumed per day was associated with a 7 percent reduction in risk of diabetes.[40] This was surprising, especially because coffee consumption, both regular and decaffeinated, has been shown to raise glucose levels after a meal; thus you would expect it to worsen diabetes, not help it.[41] The reason for the decreased diabetes risk remains uncertain, but since coffee comes from a dark-colored bean, it is likely that antioxidants, minerals, or other phytochemicals may be responsible. With this in mind, we must remember that almost all the subjects in the observational studies were eating the standard American diet and therefore were starving for antioxidants and phytochemicals.

It is most likely that the standard American diet is so nutrient-poor that a significant portion of people's phytochemical intake comes from their morning coffee! Additional studies support this possibility.[42] Chlorogenic acid and trigonelline, two of the major phytochemicals in coffee, have been shown to decrease blood glucose and insulin concentrations in the blood compared to placebos after ingesting sugar, so these phytochemicals likely increase insulin sensitivity, thereby accounting for the beneficial effects.

It is doubtful that coffee would offer any additional protection on top of a nutrient-dense diet—the responsible phytochemicals can be obtained from other plant foods and the diet would not be so lacking in antioxidants. For example, blueberries contain the antioxidant chlorogenic acid, and the phytoestrogen trigonelline is also found in peas, lentils, soybeans, and sunflower seeds. Again, the only reason that coffee is beneficial is because of the severe shortage of plant-derived phytochemicals in the diet of most Americans.

Please note: the fact that coffee is shown to have some phytochemical benefits offering a degree of protection against one disease or another does not make coffee a health food. Caffeine is still a *drug*. It is a stimulant—it gives you a false sense of increased energy, allowing you to get by with an inadequate amount of sleep. In addition to quantity of sleep, caffeine also reduces the depth of sleep. Inadequate sleep promotes disease and premature aging, and can fuel overeating behaviors. Those who drink caffeinated beverages are drawn to eat more often than necessary because they mistake caffeine withdrawal symptoms—such as shakiness, headaches, and lightheadedness—for hunger. That these detoxification symptoms are mistaken for hunger is understandable, because eating more food helps lessen them.

It is impossible to get in touch with your body's true hunger signals if you are addicted to stimulants. If you do decide to stop drinking coffee, keep in mind that it takes four to five days for the caffeine withdrawal headaches to resolve. If the symptoms are too severe, try reducing the coffee slowly. Losing weight is a more important goal for your overall health than eliminating coffee. But including caffeine does not make it easier to control your appetite and food cravings; it makes it harder.

Decaffeinated coffee is also not without risks. The chemical substances used to remove the caffeine may be hazardous. Drinking decaffeinated coffee is associated with risk of developing rheumatoid arthritis, possibly due to the caffeine-removing additives.[43] For this reason, it is probably safer to choose a water-processed decaf if you choose to drink decaffeinated coffee.

The message here is that coffee can be both good and bad, but its powerful addictive qualities, with the potential for withdrawal headaches and the potential to increase blood pressure, should make people cautious.[44] The most likely risks are almost never mentioned in news reports.

I'll say it again: coffee is a drug, not a food. And like most drugs, it may have some benefits, but its toxic effects and resultant risks may overwhelm those advantages. Caffeine is a stimulant, as noted above, and a long and healthy life is most consistently achieved when we avoid stimulants and other drugs. I do not think anyone should rely on coffee to protect against diabetes or cancer. If you do choose to drink coffee, stick to water-processed (nonchemical) decaf, and, of course, skip the doughnuts.

The Soy Debate

Asian populations have a lower incidence of hormone-related diseases, such as breast cancer, uterine cancer, and prostate cancer, than Westerners do. It has been suggested that soy consumption is one reason for this difference in disease incidence. Women who were born in Asia but migrated to the United States likewise have a lower risk of breast cancer, possibly due to their early exposure to soy. But obviously soy is only one of many factors that influence cancer risk, and now we know that it is *many* contributing factors that make a diet cancer-protective.

It is now clear that soy intake during adolescence, a time when breast tissue is most sensitive to environmental stimuli and carcinogenesis, may reduce the risk of breast cancer later in life. Recent articles in *Cancer Epidemiology* and *The American Journal of Clinical Nutrition* reported that soy consumption during childhood and teenage years reduced the risk of breast cancer in adulthood by 60 percent and 40 percent, respectively.[45]

Soybeans are rich in isoflavones, a type of phytoestrogen. Phytoestrogens are plant substances that are chemically similar to estrogen—and since higher estrogen levels promote breast cancer, some people predicted that soy would too. Now we know that the phytoestrogens in soy actually *block* the effects of the body's estrogen. Despite myths propagated on the Internet, the most recent and reliable clinical studies support a strong protective effect of minimally processed soy foods against breast cancer.

In 2006, a meta-analysis in the *Journal of the National Cancer Institute* examining data from eighteen studies on soy and breast cancer that were published between 1978 and 2004 concluded that soy overall has a protective effect.[46] Again in 2008, another meta-analysis in the *British Journal of Nutrition* compiling data from eight studies (which were not included in the 2006 meta-analysis) also concluded that soy consumption decreases breast cancer risk. These effects were dose-dependent—a

16 percent reduced risk for each 10 milligrams of soy isoflavones consumed daily.[47]

Soy has protective effects even after a diagnosis of breast cancer. A new study of breast cancer survivors has shown that premenopausal breast cancer survivors who consumed more soy had a 23 percent reduced risk of recurrence.[48]

Soy provides protection against other hormonal cancers as well. A meta-analysis of studies on soy consumption and prostate cancer found a 31 percent decrease in prostate cancer risk with a high consumption of soy foods.[49] Soy has also been shown to be protective against endometrial and ovarian cancers.[50]

Soy products such as tofu and soy milk can be useful in moving toward a plant-centered diet with less saturated fat, less animal protein, more plant protein, and more fruits and vegetables. In the United States, the majority of our soy intake, which is very low compared to that of Asian countries, is consumed via soy-based additives or isolated soy protein in processed foods.

Please note that *the most healthful soy foods are those that are minimally processed*—these include edamame, tofu, unsweetened soy milk, and tempeh. You should be aware that soy nuts and other processed soy products do not retain much of the beneficial compounds and omega-3 fats that are in the natural bean. The more the food is processed, the more these beneficial compounds are destroyed. Minimally processed soy foods are a beneficial addition to a healthy diet. I do not recommend consuming large quantities of soy products in the hopes of reducing cancer risk, however. A healthy diet should include a variety of beans, *all* of which have beneficial anticancer compounds, and not a disproportionate share of calories from soy. I always recommend the consumption of a broad variety of phytochemical-rich foods to maximize one's health. Beans are no exception—try to include various different types of beans, including soybeans.

Processed foods, because of their low nutrient levels, high amounts of salt, acrylamides, and other toxic additives, should not be considered healthy. Vegetarians and vegans who eat tofu-turkey, soy burgers, soy ice cream, soy hotdogs, soy cheese and other soy-derived processed foods on a regular basis are certainly not eating a healthy diet. Isolated soy protein is a heavily processed food with the natural micronutrients lost in processing. The key to good health is to eat *unprocessed* foods, because their nutrient-per-calorie density is high.

Omega-3 Fatty Acids

Another question I often hear is, How can I incorporate omega-3 fatty acids into my diet?

The American diet is unquestionably too low in omega-3 fats and too high in omega-6 fats. Omega-3 fats reduce inflammation, inhibit cancer development, and protect our brain and blood vessels. The basic building block of omega-3 fats is alpha-linolenic acid (ALA). ALA can be found in most nuts and seeds but is particularly abundant in flax seeds, hemp seeds, chia seeds, walnuts, and leafy green vegetables. Most people do not get enough ALA in their diet.

Among the above-listed foods, flax seeds and hemp seeds have the highest concentration of these essential fats. Besides omega-3s, these seeds also contain phytochemicals, antioxidants, and fibers that have beneficial effects to inhibit prostate, breast, and colon cancers. However, these protective nutrients and cancer-fighting lignans are not present in significant quantities in the *oil,* only in the whole *seed.* Flax seeds are best ground to a fine powder before use because they are difficult to chew and thus may pass through undigested. Once the seeds are ground, store them in the freezer to preserve freshness.

The short-chain omega-3 fats found in seeds, nuts, and greens are the building blocks of the longer-chain DHA fat that our bodies need for proper functioning of our brain, nervous system, and immune system. Besides our own body's production from ALA, we also get EPA and DHA from fish, fish oil, and algae.

Greens, walnuts, and seeds supply ALA

$$ALA \longrightarrow EPA \longrightarrow DHA$$

Fish and algae supply EPA and DHA

In the past, fish or fish oil was thought to be the only source of EPA and DHA, but recently EPA and DHA have become available via a vegan source extracted from omega-3-containing algae grown indoors in clean and controlled conditions.

We do not need *lots* of EPA and DHA, but problems may arise when people become deficient in these needed fats. Low EPA and DHA levels have been associated with:

- Heart disease

- Depression

- Cancer

- Anxiety/panic

- Alzheimer's disease

- Hyperactivity

- Attention deficit disorder

- Allergies

- Autoimmune illnesses

- Dermatologic disorders

- Inflammatory bowel disease

Scientists have known for many years that humans can convert short-chain omega-3 fats (ALA) from seeds and greens into the valuable EPA and DHA. The question is, Can we achieve optimal levels without the consumption of fish? Studies show that people have varying ability to convert ALA into DHA, so the answer is ambiguous: some people ingesting ALA from greens, flax, and walnuts can achieve adequate levels of EPA and DHA, while others do not manufacture optimal amounts.[51] Men generally convert less than women, and the ability to convert declines with aging, suggesting that supplements may be more important for older males.

Fish are rich in omega-3s, but fish are concentrated animal protein and accumulate environmental pollutants. Eating too much animal protein raises IGF-1 levels, as we saw, which in turn are linked to cancer.[52] Regarding pollutants in fish, the Environmental Protection Agency warns primarily of mercury, PCBs, chlordane, dioxins, and DDT. High levels of PCBs, chlordane, and dioxins detected in body fat have been associated with threefold to tenfold increases in the occurrence of cancer.[53] The dumping of toxic waste into our oceans has definitely taken a toll. So while DHA is definitely a beneficial fat, we have to reconsider the source in which we find it.

Since fish are highly polluted compared to other foods, we have to take a closer look at the typical recommendations of health authorities to consume more fish. Increasing fish consumption was found to be linked to a modest increase in the incidence of diabetes as well as increased risk of prostate cancer and breast cancer in some studies.[54]

After many years of reviewing the evidence and recording mercury levels in patients—levels that invariably correlate well with their fish consumption—I recommend consuming little or no fish and strongly advise against consuming any of those species of fish notoriously high in mercury, such as shark, swordfish, mackerel, pike, and bluefish.

Note, too, that the amount of DHA can vary significantly depending on the fish and the location. Farm-raised fish such as tilapia has none, and even some salmon (especially farm-raised) has very little DHA.

If you avoid fish and instead consume fish oil, you may still have a problem. One problem with fish oil is that much of the fat has already turned rancid. If you have ever cut open a capsule and tasted it, you may have found that it can taste like gasoline. Many people complain of burping, indigestion, and fish breath. I have also observed that rancidity of fish oil places a stress on the liver and can even cause abnormalities in liver function. If using fish oil, make sure it is purified and certified to be free of mercury, and cut at least one capsule open and taste the oil directly, to make sure it does not taste rotten.

Not everyone requires supplementation with EPA and DHA. A person's specific need can be ascertained with a blood test, but since this test is not universally available, most of us can assure nutritional adequacy of EPA and DHA without using fish oil, by just adding a small amount of a vegan EPA or DHA supplement. Today, laboratory-cultivated DHA is available that is made, as noted above, from algae grown indoors, free of the pollutants found in algae collected in the wild—that is, without mercury or other toxins. Recently a randomized, placebo-controlled study showed that 100 milligrams of DHA daily increased the omega-3 index from 4.8 (poor) to 8.4 (optimal) percent, demonstrating that even a relatively low dose of pure DHA taken daily is as effective as a much higher amount of fish oil.[55]

Cancer is a complex disease, and when we consider the overall picture, we should be cautious with any supplementation, including that of omega-3 fats. More than needed may not be better when it comes to omega-3 fatty acids. However, a deficiency of nutrients the body requires is never favorable for health.

In conclusion, to assure omega-3 adequacy, unless blood tests demonstrate otherwise, I recommend 100 to 200 milligrams a day of DHA, plus 1 tablespoon of ground flax seeds for ALA. Bear in mind: *all* nutrients can be harmful in deficiency or excess.

Organic Fruits and Vegetables and the Dangers of Pesticides

The Environmental Protection Agency reports that the majority of pesticides now in use are probable or possible cancer causes. Studies of farmworkers who work with pesticides suggest a link between pesticide use and brain cancer, Parkinson's disease, multiple myeloma, leukemia, lymphoma, and cancers of the stomach and prostate.[56]

The question remains, however: Does the low level of pesticides remaining on our food after harvest present much of a risk?

Previously, the large number of studies performed on the typical pesticide-treated produce demonstrated that consumption of produce, whether organic or not, is related to lower rates of cancer and increased disease protection. This suggested that the health benefits of eating phytochemical-rich produce greatly outweighed any risks that pesticide residues might pose. As such, some scientists argue that the extremely low levels of pesticide residue remaining on produce is insignificant and that there are naturally occurring toxins in all natural foods that are more significant.

This viewpoint may no longer be wholly accurate: recent studies have documented a link between pesticides ingested from foods and certain diseases. Organophosphate exposure (organophosphate pesticides are used on several crops, including corn, apples, pears, grapes, berries, and peaches) has been associated with ADHD, behavior problems, and neurodevelopmental deficits in children.[57] A number of pesticides may have damaging effects on the brain that contribute to Parkinson's disease, including rotenone and paraquat, which are used on a variety of vegetable crops, and organochlorines, which are now found primarily in fatty foods like meat, dairy, and fish (having found their way up the food chain after an initial application on vegetation).[58]

If you are concerned about pesticides and chemicals, keep in mind that animal products, such as dairy, fish, and beef, contain the most toxic chemical residues. Because cows and steers eat large amounts of tainted feed, certain pesticides and dangerous chemicals are found in higher concentrations in animal foods. Nevertheless, by centering your diet on unrefined plant foods, you will automatically reduce your exposure to the majority of dangerous chemicals.

It is better to eat fruits and vegetables grown and harvested using pesticides than to not eat them at all; but it is also wise to minimize your pesticide exposure. The Environmental Working Group provides a list of produce called the "Dirty Dozen" (those highest in pesticides) and the "Clean Fifteen" (lowest in pesticides). These are their most recent lists.

HIGHEST IN PESTICIDES— BUY ORGANIC IF POSSIBLE	LOWEST IN PESTICIDES— BUY EITHER ORGANIC OR CONVENTIONAL
Celery	Onion
Peaches	Avocado
Strawberries	Sweet corn
Apples	Pineapple
Blueberries	Mango
Nectarines	Sweet peas
Bell peppers	Asparagus
Spinach	Kiwi
Kale	Cabbage
Cherries	Eggplant
Potatoes	Cantaloupe
Grapes (imported)	Watermelon
	Grapefruit
	Sweet potato
	Honeydew melon

It makes sense to peel fruits, if possible, and not to eat potato skins, unless you are able to purchase those vegetables in organic form. Remove and discard the outermost leaves of lettuce and cabbage, if not organically grown; and other surfaces that cannot be peeled can be washed with soap and water, or a commercial vegetable wash.

When we buy organic, we minimize our pesticide exposure, and we also minimize the amount of these pesticides that our environment is exposed to. Organic farming is clearly the more environmentally friendly choice. According to the U.S. Department of Agriculture, organic farming "integrates cultural, biological, and mechanical practices that foster cycling of resources, promote ecological balance, and conserve biodiversity."[59] Supporting organic agriculture increases the demand for organic produce and decreases the percentage of farmland (and farmworkers) exposed to potentially harmful agricultural chemicals.

Organic produce usually has more nutrients—especially minerals and antioxidant nutrients—than conventional produce. Organic apples, plums, blueberries, grapes, strawberries, and corn have all been shown to have higher antioxidant capacities than their conventional counterparts. Similarly, organic strawberries were found to have more anticancer activity than conventional strawberries.[60]

Scientists have theorized that when the plants are grown without pesticides, they are forced to deal with the stress of insects, which causes them to produce more of those antioxidant compounds that are beneficial to humans.

Bottom line: buying organic is a wise choice—organic foods taste better, and organic agriculture protects farmers and our environment.

Super Immunity and Autoimmune Disease

When our immune system is working as intended, it serves as our inner army, defending our lives and protecting us all the time. However, after years of nutritional abuse it can not only lose its protective function (by which it attacks microbes and tumor cells), but can actually attack *normal* cells. When our immune system attacks our skin, joints, and internal organs, we have what is called an "autoimmune" disease. Psoriasis, lupus, rheumatoid arthritis, and connective tissue disease are examples, but there are about a hundred clinical syndromes considered autoimmune diseases. Inflammatory bowel diseases, such as Crohn's and ulcerative colitis, are also autoimmune diseases. They are in a class distinct from the others, however: they are not typically classified as "rheumatologic," as the others are, because they are typically treated by gastroenterologists, not rheumatologists. Nevertheless, they are likewise diseases where inflammatory markers are visible in the blood and are of the same class as systemic autoimmune disorders.

I have been successfully treating and reporting positive outcomes in patients with autoimmune diseases through nutritional intervention for more than twenty years.[61] In a recent survey of members at DrFuhrman.com, sixteen individuals with rheumatoid arthritis responded. All of them reported significant improvement in symptoms, and half of them reported complete resolution of symptoms. Obviously, not every patient with these diseases can make a complete, drug-free recovery. However, the amazing thing is that my experience enables me to assure patients with a reasonable degree of certainty that their condition will likely improve and in many cases resolve.

It is not just *my* findings that document improvement in autoimmune conditions with good nutrition. Vegetable-based and vegan diets have been reported to be effective against autoimmune disease in the medical literature.[62] I find that not just opting for a vegan diet, but also improving the diet with foods rich in immune-supporting micronutrients, and especially green cruciferous vegetables, adds further potential for recovery. A diet high in micronutrients and antioxidants is a key to repairing immune system defects that may lead to disease.[63]

The human body's complicated immune response is controlled with a system of checks and balances, just like our democratic government. Many components are involved in this immune-mediated attack. First, our antibodies label areas worthy of attack; then other cells work to call out the alarm-secreting substances that attract and promote proliferation of other attacking cells. Finally, there are cells that control the attack, modify it, and turn it off at the precise moment to prevent an excessive response. In autoimmune disorders such as lupus, we have an immune response that reacts in an uncontrolled fashion—a response that is not properly immuno-regulated.

As our understanding of the mechanism and causes of inflammation increases, so does our ability to understand the factors that create a favorable environment for improvement and healing of autoimmune disease. The scientific basis for the nutritional treatment of autoimmune disease hinges on the removal of toxins and food excesses, while at the same time supplying a high level of nutritional factors that help normalize a malfunctioning immune response that overreacts to stimuli and does not shut off.

Despite excellent clinical results and the publication of case studies and medical journal articles documenting favorable outcomes with nutritional interventions,[64] medical authorities and major research centers are not interested in studying nutritional excellence as a therapy for rheumatologic diseases.

It is difficult to move against an entrenched status quo that utilizes and tests medications as the only option. If my approach to autoimmune illness were taught in medical schools and residency programs, primary care physicians could begin this nutritional approach at the earliest signs of autoimmune illness with their patients, instead of prescribing a lifetime of medications with dangerous side effects. I am presently working with the Nutritional Research Project at nutritionalresearch .org to see that these more comprehensive studies come to fruition.

The successes I have seen in my years of practice are compelling. Consider the following account:

> I had lupus for twenty years. I took Plaquenil, Methotrexate, Prednisone, and other toxic drugs in high dosages and still lived my life

imprisoned in isolation and pain with many lost years. I searched on the Web for years, looking for something else. Over the years, I had done acupuncture, chiropractic, massage, exercise, stress management, vitamins, herbs, various oils, including fish oils, antibiotics, and other treatments. I am so grateful to have found Dr. Fuhrman. Thanks to him, today I have a normal life, full of energy, the joint pain is gone, and I am on no medication.

—Cheryl Platt

Typically, patients come to see me with lupus or rheumatoid arthritis and tell a similar story. Their doctor typically gets mad if patients even suggest a natural approach to their problem. Debra Black's story below is typical:

I had been feeling fatigued and a little achy for a few months. And then, after being referred to a dermatologist for a rash on my face, I was told I had lupus. With hardly a discussion about it, the dermatologist wrote out a prescription for Plaquenil and Prednisone. I questioned the doctor about the risks of the drugs and was told I would need them for the rest of my life, and if I did not take them the lupus could then attack my joints and kidneys, and even kill me. I left the office in tears.

I then went to see Dr. Fuhrman, looking for another way. He told me about his success in treating lupus with nutritional therapy and was confident he could help me. He pointed to a few medical studies that supported the effectiveness of this type of treatment, but he said most doctors are simply not interested in anything but drugs.

I had nothing to lose. I followed Dr. Fuhrman's vegetable-based diet with his blended salads, fresh vegetable juices, vegetable/bean soups with onions and mushrooms, and added cruciferous greens and lots of berries and seeds. He taught me how to make his delicious soups too. He had me take three separate nutritional supplements and wrote out a plan for me, telling me exactly what to eat and what not to eat. I followed it like a champ.

Within six days after beginning Dr. Fuhrman's program I felt "freaky," like there was a sunburn inside my entire body. My skin was warm, itchy. I called Dr. Fuhrman in a panic. He was pleased; he said that this is a great sign to be occurring so soon and that my body was withdrawing from my prior toxic diet and detoxifying. He explained that this was the first step before my ugly skin rash could heal. Within a few more days my stiffness and pain had improved significantly. I couldn't believe I felt so good, so fast. Within one month, the discoid (lupus-caused) skin rash had disappeared. I looked and felt radiant. Everyone commented on how good I looked. My skin looked soft and smooth; I was well again. I went back to the dermatologist, excited to share my story, and he became irate and screamed at me—ridiculous nonsense he said, and told me to get out of his office.

Achieving superior health via nutritional excellence gives a person with an autoimmune disorder the only opportunity for a complete, drug-free remission. In many cases a vegetarian diet alone helps substantially. It is important to keep in mind that food is our major contact with the external environment, and food choices can negatively or positively modulate the immune system. In addition to inherently toxic substances that may be ingested, partially digested animal proteins can be absorbed into the bloodstream, playing a significant role in promoting an excessive antibody response and thus contributing to autoimmune diseases.

However, in most cases more specific dietary modifications along with nutritional supplements are required to maximize the therapeutic response. Over the last fifteen years, having treated and helped hundreds of patients with autoimmune disease, I have found that the greatest percentage of patients achieve excellent results if they utilize a high-nutrient dietary program rich in greens—especially the cruciferous vegetables, such as cabbage, broccoli, and kale—in conjunction with some helpful nutritional supplements.

The autoimmune protocol has some important features:

1. High-nutrient vegan diet, rich in green vegetables

2. Blended salads and/or vegetable juices (utilizing leafy greens) to increase absorption of favorable phytochemical compounds

3. Supplementation with EPA and DHA[65]

4. Supplementation with beneficial bowel flora

5. Supplementation with natural anti-inflammatory substances such as turmeric, ginger, quercetin, and other bioflavonoids

6. Supplementation with a multivitamin/multimineral, plus additional vitamin D[66]

7. Dietary avoidance of salt, wheat, oil, and concentrated sweets

The ability to achieve substantial improvement and even complete remission of these supposedly incurable illnesses is exciting. Patients with these conditions are typically highly motivated to get well and amenable to any health-supporting changes that may facilitate their recovery. I know that there are many thousands of people who visit their doctors begging for a nontoxic natural approach to getting well and are told that diet and nutritional interventions do not work.

Jill's story is typical of those of so many other suffering individuals:

My lupus story began in 1992, when I was thirty-two years old. I had experienced severe joint pains, fatigue, and a red facial rash. The blood tests came back specific for lupus. At first I thought this was good news—a diagnosis, now we can do something about it. Well, I was then told there is no cure and I would have to live with it and take medication for the rest of my life. I was even told by the rheumatologist that I might die from it. Even with the medications, I had a constant low-grade fever, low energy, a bright red face, stiffness, and joint pain.

I could not accept this death sentence and a life dependent on toxic drugs. I researched everything I could find about this disease and tried changing to a vegetarian diet and alternative medicine with some degree of success. I lived in Virginia and took a train trip up to New Jersey to visit Dr. Fuhrman. I was convinced to take the next step to regain my health and decided to adopt a healthier, "whole foods diet" and do some fasting. Soon I felt like a teenager again; my face was cool and white for the first time in years, my joints felt great, and I had lots of energy. I lost a little weight and looked great.

I went back to visit my rheumatologist, who was on staff at a teaching hospital. I just knew he was going to be interested in my story and recovery from lupus. When I started to tell him of my experience and my newfound good health, he wrote "spontaneous recovery" in the chart. I was shocked. He was not the least bit interested in hearing the details of my recovery, and practically walked out of the room when I started to explain what happened.

Now, nine years later, I remain free from the symptoms of lupus. Lupus is no longer part of my life. I play tennis and compete on a local team. No one who knows me today would ever guess that I used to be in so much pain that I couldn't even shake someone's hand.

No matter where your health is today, you can improve it. When we make the right choices, we can live better and be healthier. Do not be complacent with doing what other people do. Do not be complacent with taking medications for the rest of your life. You can recover. Your body has an amazing healing potential waiting to be unleashed by the gift of superior nutrition.

Achieving superior health is well within your reach. And in the process, you will look better, feel better, and live longer. Better still, Super Immunity can be delicious, as you will see in the following pages.

CHAPTER SEVEN

Menus
and Recipes

*When my child was 18 months old and suffering from his
fourth ear infection and fourth course of antibiotics, my
search for a better solution led me to Dr. Fuhrman. After one
visit, we changed my son's diet according to Dr. Fuhrman's
instructions and Evan never suffered another ear infection.*

—Ondria Westfall

To really experience all the pleasures and benefits that a micro-nutrient-rich Super Immunity diet has to offer, you must learn to make nutrient-rich meals in your own kitchen. To show you the concepts in action, and give you a feel for the delicious flavors and textures of nutrient-rich food, I have provided two weeks of sample meal plans and an assortment of delicious recipes. These will help you understand and master the basic techniques and principles of high-nutrient food preparation.

A good place to start is with salads. Make sure you and your family eat a big green salad at least once a day. Since salad is so important, the unique healthy and tasty salad dressings below are the most important recipes. You must try them to see how good they taste.

If you feel that these recommendations are too daunting to implement all at once, at first simply make sure that both lunch and dinner include either a salad or a cooked green vegetable (and add mushrooms and onions to that vegetable most days).

The next step after that is to make a big pot of one of the vegetable-bean soups at least once a week. After your initial meal, you'll be able to use it the rest of the week as leftovers.

Within two weeks you could accomplish these basics: a salad every day, a bowl of veggie-bean soup with mushrooms and onions most days, and cooked greens every day. But that's just the beginning: you may find, after trying many of the fantastic recipes I have provided here, that your fears of change are overcome by pleasure and the enjoyment of great food.

You can switch around foods and adjust the recipes to reflect your own tastes and lifestyle. Except for people who employ their own cook, hardly anybody prepares different dishes like this on a daily basis. In the real world, you make enough of one dish to cover multiple meals and then don't cook for a few days, until all the leftovers are eaten. So in reality, these two weeks of recipes should actually give you a complete variety of dishes to use for many more weeks.

You can eat simply and enjoy fruit and nuts for breakfast, a big salad with beans and a healthy dressing for lunch, and then a nice bowl of soup with dinner that was (made a few days earlier). Life is busy. When you cook, *do* make enough to enjoy leftovers for several days. Soups can last up to five days in the refrigerator or even longer if you freeze them. Salad dressings will last three days refrigerated and still taste fresh. So if you are cooking for a family, double the size of the recipes supplied here so they'll last for more than one meal.

Plan your cooking and shopping schedule so you have some evenings where you know there will be no need for cooking; then you can plan other fun family activities or exercise on those nights. Many people find that shopping twice a week and cooking twice a week is adequate to prepare most of the healthy dishes they need for the full week.

Remember, you can eat as much as you want of raw and cooked vegetables and fresh fruits. Include a serving of beans in your diet each day, and at least 1 ounce of raw nuts and seeds (about ¼ cup). Since you are giving up lots of unhealthy foods, treat yourself to plenty of delicious and exotic fruits and vegetables and a delicious healthy dessert after dinner. Try different fresh herbs and spices to season your foods.

Always keep a good assortment of healthy food in the house; and when you leave the house for work, travel, or leisure, pack up food to take with you so that you are not stranded with unhealthy choices. The key to eating healthfully is to stock your house with a good variety of healthy foods, cook up delicious healthy recipes, and remove unhealthy food choices from your home.

As noted above, I have included a number of healthy salad dressing recipes to be used with your own combination of greens. There are also a variety of salad recipes that include both dressing and suggested vegetables for the salad, but mix and match the dressings and make your own creations. These recipes are designed to give you a delicious *start;* with experience, you can modify them for variety and your own preferences.

A small amount of animal products can be added to any vegetable or bean dish for a different flavor, if desired. However, I suggest that you keep the animal product additions well below 10 ounces for a female and 12 ounces for a male for the entire week. In other words, don't eat a large portion of animal products at any meal, but use such products in condiment or flavoring amounts to add taste to a soup, stew, or salad. You will note, through following and eating some of these recipes, that a very small amount of meat, fish, or seafood per serving can add a familiar flavor. Completely avoid processed, cured, or barbecued meats.

The use of animal products in a nutritarian diet is optional, as we have seen; one can be vegan, near-vegan, or flexitarian, using animal products semiregularly but in very small amounts, and in all of these iting healthfully. If you want to use animal products in your diet to retain that flavor, restrict your consumption of oil and other processed foods even more so that you still have high-nutrient produce forming 90 percent of your caloric intake. To keep animal products appropriately limited in your diet, I suggest that if you use some on a particular day, make the next day completely vegan. That way you will easily not exceed the low levels I prescribe for Super Immunity and an anticancer lifestyle.

All the recipes in this book are delicious and complete as vegan recipes. For some of the recipes, however, I suggest a nonvegan option for those who want to use a small amount of animal product to enhance the taste. It's your choice. For example, you may serve the Thai Longevity Stew with some small chunks of cooked shrimp or scallop mixed in. The Creamy Cruciferous Curry may be flavored with shredded strips of chicken, turkey, or rattlesnake (kidding!). All recipes that have a nonvegan option are identified with an asterisk below and are listed on page 188.

Super Immunity Menu Plans

Week 1

DAY 1

Breakfast

Forbidden Rice Pudding

Lunch

Spinach Salad with Strawberry Sesame Vinaigrette

Tangy White Beans and Zucchini

Dinner

Raw veggies (snow peas, broccoli, and carrots) with Island Black Bean Dip

Braised Kale and Squash with Pumpkin Seeds

Black Cherry Sorbet

DAY 2

Breakfast

    Detox Green Tea

    Super Seed Oatmeal

Lunch

    Aztec Stuffer

    Sliced avocado

    Pineapple or other fresh fruit

Dinner

    Shiitake Watercress Soup*

    Super Food Stuffed Peppers

    Chia Cookies and Almond Hemp Nutri-Milk

DAY 3

Breakfast

    Purple Power Smoothie

Lunch

    Shiitake Watercress Soup* (leftover)

    Acorn Squash Supreme

    Watermelon or other fresh fruit

Dinner

    Salad of mixed greens with assorted veggies and ground chia seeds
      with Banana Ginger Dressing

    Creamy Cruciferous Curry*

    Mango or other fresh fruit

DAY 4

Breakfast

Wild Blueberry Hot Breakfast

Lunch

Caesar's Secret Salad

Berry Boost Gelatin

Dinner

Seasoned Kale Chips and Popcorn

Dr. Fuhrman's Famous Anticancer Soup

Strawberries with Chocolate Dip

DAY 5

Breakfast

Quick Banana Berry Breakfast to Go

Lunch

Salad of baby greens with Orange Cashame Dressing

Dr. Fuhrman's Famous Anticancer Soup (leftover)

Kiwi or other fresh fruit

Dinner

Salad of mixed greens and arugula topped with sunflower seeds
with Russian Vinaigrette Dressing

Mighty Mushroom Stroganoff* over whole-wheat pasta

Fresh or frozen cherries

DAY 6

Breakfast

Waldorf Blended Salad

Lunch

Italian Stuffer*

Sliced tomato sprinkled with balsamic vinegar and Mediterranean
pine nuts

Melon or other fresh fruit

Dinner

Triple Treat Cabbage Salad

Goji Chili Stew

Apple Berrynut Bites

DAY 7

Breakfast

Veggie Scramble*

Almond Hemp Nutri-Milk

Lunch

Tomato Bisque

Marinated Kale Salad

Sliced apples with Golden Onion Morsels

Dinner

Endive spears and romaine leaves with Black Bean and Corn Salsa

Better Burgers* with avocado, lettuce, tomato, and red onion on
whole-grain buns

Home-Style Ketchup

Steamed broccoli

Healthy Chocolate Cake

Week 2

DAY 1

Breakfast

    Sweet Beet Potato Cakes with Strawberry Sauce

Lunch

    Salad of romaine lettuce and napa cabbage with Goji Balsamic Dressing

    Cremini Ratatouille

    Clementines or other fresh fruit

Dinner

    Lisa's Lovely Lentil Stew

    Green Leafy Moroccan Medley

    Fresh pineapple chunks

DAY 2

Breakfast

    Go Berry Breakfast Bars

    Cinnamon Apple Omega Milk

Lunch

    Mumbai Stuffer

    Carrot and red pepper sticks

    Papaya with lime or other fresh fruit

Dinner

    Salad of mixed greens and tomato with Pesto Dressing

    "Cheesy" Kale Soup

    Fresh or frozen blueberries

DAY 3

Breakfast

Very Berry Smoothie

Lunch

Eggplant Hummus

Raw vegetables (zucchini, red peppers, snap peas)

Portobello Mushrooms and Beans

Cherries or other fresh fruit

Dinner

Apple Bok Choy Salad

Swiss Chard and Sweet Potato Gratin*

Golden Delicious Truffles

DAY 4

Breakfast

Phyto-Blast Breakfast Bowl

Lunch

Creamy Butternut Squash Soup with Mushrooms

Black Bean Lettuce Bundles

Tropical Fruit Salad

Dinner

Nutri-Green Salad with Black Fig Dressing

Thai Longevity Stew*

Wild Blueberry Apple Pie or mixed berries

DAY 5

Breakfast

Pomegranate Muesli

Lunch

Powerhouse Micro Salad

Apples with raw cashew butter

Dinner

Spaghetti Squash Primavera

All-American Spinach with Mushrooms

Black Bean Brownies

DAY 6

Breakfast

Got Greens Smoothie

Lunch

Easy Vegetable Pizza*

Brussels Sprouts Polonaise

Grapes or other fresh fruit

Dinner

Salad of mixed greens and broccoli sprouts with Peanut Ginger
Dressing

Golden Austrian Cauliflower Cream Soup

Chunky Blueberry Walnut Sorbet

DAY 7

Breakfast

Blackberry Apple Surprise

Lunch

Rainbow Chopped Salad

Golden Austrian Cauliflower Cream Soup (leftover)

Mango or other fresh fruit

Dinner

Raw vegetables (cucumber, endive spears, red pepper)

Simple Guacamole

Bean Enchiladas

Low-sodium salsa

Coconut Carrot Cream Pie

Recipe Index

Breakfast

Blackberry Apple Surprise   189
Forbidden Rice Pudding   190
Go Berry Breakfast Bars   191
Phyto-Blast Breakfast Bowl   191
Pomegranate Muesli   192
Quick Banana Berry Breakfast to Go   192
Super Seed Oatmeal   193
Sweet Beet Potato Cakes with Strawberry Sauce   194
Veggie Scramble   195
Wild Blueberry Hot Breakfast   195

Smoothies, Blended Salads, and Other Drinks

Almond Hemp Nutri-Milk   196
Cinnamon Apple Omega Milk   196
Detox Green Tea   197
Got Greens Smoothie   197
Purple Power Smoothie   198
Very Berry Smoothie   198
Waldorf Blended Salad   198

Salad Dressings

Banana Ginger Dressing   199
Goji Balsamic Dressing   199
Orange Cashame Dressing   200
Peanut Ginger Dressing   200
Pesto Dressing   201
Russian Vinaigrette Dressing   201

Salads

Apple Bok Choy Salad 202
Caesar's Secret Salad 203
Marinated Kale Salad 204
Nutri-Green Salad with Black Fig Dressing 205
Powerhouse Micro Salad 206
Rainbow Chopped Salad 206
Spinach Salad with Strawberry Sesame Vinaigrette 207
Triple Treat Cabbage Salad 208
Tropical Fruit Salad 209

Dips, Snacks, and Condiments

Black Bean and Corn Salsa 210
Eggplant Hummus 211
Golden Onion Morsels 211
Home-Style Ketchup 212
Island Black Bean Dip 212
Seasoned Kale Chips and Popcorn 213
Simple Guacamole 213

Soups

"Cheesy" Kale Soup 214
Creamy Butternut Squash Soup with Mushrooms 215
Dr. Fuhrman's Famous Anticancer Soup 216
Golden Austrian Cauliflower Cream Soup 217
Shiitake Watercress Soup 218
Tomato Bisque 219

Main Dishes

Acorn Squash Supreme 220
All-American Spinach with Mushrooms 220
Bean Enchiladas 221

Better Burgers   222

Black Bean Lettuce Bundles   223

Braised Kale and Squash with Pumpkin Seeds   224

Brussels Sprouts Polonaise   224

Creamy Cruciferous Curry   225

Cremini Ratatouille   226

Easy Vegetable Pizza   226

Goji Chili Stew   227

Green Leafy Moroccan Medley   228

Lisa's Lovely Lentil Stew   229

Mighty Mushroom Stroganoff   230

Portobello Mushrooms and Beans   231

Spaghetti Squash Primavera   232

Super Food Stuffed Peppers   233

Swiss Chard and Sweet Potato Gratin   234

Tangy White Beans and Zucchini   235

Thai Longevity Stew   236

Pita/Wrap Stuffers

Aztec Stuffer   237

Italian Stuffer   237

Mumbai Stuffer   237

Desserts

Apple Berrynut Bites   238

Berry Boost Gelatin   238

Black Bean Brownies   239

Black Cherry Sorbet   239

Chia Cookies   240

Chocolate Dip with Fresh Fruit and Berries   240

Chunky Blueberry Walnut Sorbet   241

Coconut Carrot Cream Pie   242

Golden Delicious Truffles   243
Healthy Chocolate Cake   244
Wild Blueberry Apple Pie   245

Recipes with Nonvegan Options

Better Burgers   222
Creamy Cruciferous Curry   225
Easy Vegetable Pizza   226
Italian Stuffer   237
Mighty Mushroom Stroganoff   230
Shiitake Watercress Soup   218
Swiss Chard and Sweet Potato Gratin   234
Thai Longevity Stew   236
Veggie Scramble   195

BREAKFAST RECIPES

Several of the recipes below contain Dr. Fuhrman's Black Fig Vinegar, Dr. Fuhrman's Blood Orange Vinegar, Dr. Fuhrman's Riesling Raisin Vinegar, Dr. Fuhrman's VegiZest, and/or Dr. Fuhrman's MatoZest. I include these premixed options, available at DrFuhrman.com or fine health food stores, for your convenience; however, the recipes can be made without them. If you use one of the alternate ingredients that I suggest in a recipe, start with a small amount and add more according to your own taste, as the intensity of spice products can differ markedly from brand to brand.

Blackberry Apple Surprise

Serves: 4

    1 cup currants
    ⅓ cup water
    8 apples, peeled, cored, and diced
    ½ cup blackberries
    ½ cup chopped walnuts
    4 tablespoons ground flax seeds
    1 tablespoon ground cinnamon
    1 teaspoon vanilla extract

Place the currants on the bottom of a medium saucepan and add the water. Place the diced apples on top. Cover and steam over very low heat for 5 minutes. Add the blackberries and cook for 2 more minutes. Transfer the apple-blackberry mixture to a bowl and mix well with remaining ingredients.

Forbidden Rice Pudding

Serves: 4

2 cups cooked black rice
2 cups unsweetened soy, hemp, or almond milk
½ cup dried apple, soaked in ½ cup water until soft, then diced
(reserve soaking water to use in recipe)
1 cup frozen wild blueberries
2 Medjool dates (or 4 Deglet Noor), pitted and finely chopped
1 tablespoon currants
2 teaspoons ground cinnamon
2 teaspoons vanilla extract
1 tablespoon ground chia seeds

Place all ingredients, except chia seeds, in a medium-size pot. Bring to a boil over medium-high heat; then reduce heat to simmer on low for 15 minutes. Turn off the heat and add the chia seeds and stir well, letting the mixture sit covered for another 5 minutes.

Great for breakfast or for dinner dessert, served warm or cold, with a dollop of whipped frozen banana cream on top.

Make the frozen banana cream by blending frozen banana slices with a small amount to vanilla hemp milk or vanilla soy milk.

Go Berry Breakfast Bars

Serves: 8

1 ripe banana
1 cup old-fashioned rolled oats (not quick or instant)
1 cup frozen blueberries, thawed
¼ cup raisins
⅛ cup pomegranate juice
2 tablespoons finely chopped dates
1 tablespoon chopped walnuts
1 tablespoon goji berries
1 tablespoon raw sunflower seeds
2 tablespoons ground flax seeds

Preheat oven to 350°F. Mash peeled banana in a large bowl. Add remaining ingredients and mix thoroughly. Lightly wipe an 8 x 8–inch baking pan with a small amount of olive oil. Spread mixture in pan. Bake for 25 minutes. Cool on wire rack and cut into bars. Refrigerate any leftover bars.

Phyto-Blast Breakfast Bowl

Serves: 2

1 apple, cored and sliced
1 banana, sliced
1 orange, sectioned
½ cup blueberries
½ cup sliced strawberries
2 tablespoons ground chia, hemp, or flax seeds
2 tablespoons chopped walnuts

Combine fruit and berries. Add seeds and nuts and toss.

Pomegranate Muesli
Serves: 2

    ½ cup pomegranate juice
    ¼ cup steel-cut or old-fashioned rolled oats (not quick or instant)
    1 apple, peeled, cored, and grated
    4 raw cashews or hazelnuts, coarsely chopped
    ½ cup halved grapes
    ½ cup cubed cantaloupe
    ½ cup sliced fresh strawberries
    1 tablespoon currants
    1 tablespoon ground flax seeds

Soak oats in pomegranate juice overnight in refrigerator. Oats will absorb the liquid. In the morning, combine oats with remaining ingredients.

Note: You may add or substitute any fruits according to taste.

Quick Banana Berry Breakfast to Go
Serves: 2

    2 cups fresh or frozen blueberries
    2 bananas, sliced
    ½ cup old-fashioned rolled oats (not quick or instant)
    ⅓ cup pomegranate juice
    2 tablespoons chopped walnuts
    1 tablespoon raw sunflower seeds
    2 tablespoons dried currants

Combine all ingredients in a small microwave-proof bowl. Heat in the microwave for 3 minutes.

Alternatively, you can combine all ingredients, unheated, in a sealed container and eat later, either hot or cold.

Super Seed Oatmeal

Serves: 2

1 cup old-fashioned rolled oats (not quick or instant)
1½ cups unsweetened vanilla soy, hemp, or almond milk
1 apple, peeled, cored, and chopped
1 cup frozen blueberries or mixed berries, thawed
¼ cup raisins
1 tablespoon raw sunflower seeds
1 tablespoon ground flax seeds
1 tablespoon ground hemp seeds
½ teaspoon ground cinnamon

Cook oats according to package directions, using soy milk instead of water. Mix remaining ingredients together and stir into the oats.

Sweet Beet Potato Cakes with Strawberry Sauce
Makes: 12 cakes

For the Cakes:
- 1 pound sweet potatoes, cut into big chunks
- 2 large beets, cut into big chunks
- 2 cups sliced mushrooms
- 3 cups very finely chopped collard greens
- 1 medium onion, diced
- 1 tablespoon Dijon mustard
- 1 tablespoon Dr. Fuhrman's Black Fig Vinegar or balsamic vinegar
- 1 tablespoon fresh chopped dill
- 1 tablespoon ground chia seeds

For the Strawberry Sauce:
- 1 apple, peeled, cored, and diced
- 1 cup frozen strawberries
- ½ cup dried apple slices
- ½ cup water
- 2 tablespoons Dr. Fuhrman's Black Fig Vinegar or balsamic vinegar
- 1 tablespoon Dijon mustard

Place the sweet potatoes and beets together in a covered pot and steam for 20–30 minutes until fork-tender. Set aside to cool. When the sweet potatoes and beets are cool, remove the skins and mash.

Sauté the onion in a pan in 3 tablespoons water for a few minutes until it is translucent and tender. Add the mushrooms and collard greens and continue to cook and stir with a wooden spatula another 5 minutes, until all the vegetables are tender. Add this mixture to a bowl with the sweet potatoes and beets and add the mustard, vinegar, dill, and ground chia seeds. Mix well and then form into patties. Bake at very low heat (200°F) for 2 hours, which dehydrates and hardens the cakes or patties.

To make strawberry sauce, place the fresh apple, strawberries, and dried apple in a small pot with the water. Bring to a boil over medium-high heat; then reduce heat and simmer, covered, for 20 minutes. Mash with a potato masher or blend to desired consistency.

Serve potato cakes with sauce.

Veggie Scramble

Serves: 2

> 3 cups baby spinach
> 1 cup chopped onion
> 1 cup chopped green pepper
> 1 cup diced tomatoes
> ½ block firm tofu
> ¼ cup unsweetened soy, hemp, or almond milk
> 1 tablespoon Dr. Fuhrman's VegiZest or other no-salt seasoning
>   mix, adjusted to taste

Sauté spinach, onion, pepper, and tomatoes in a bit of water until tender. Squeeze out as much water as you can from the tofu and then crumble it over the vegetable mixture; cook the combined mixture, stirring occasionally, until tofu is lightly browned. Add seasoning, if desired.

Nonvegan option: This recipe can be made with 3 eggs and ¼ cup unsweetened soy, hemp, or almond milk instead of tofu. Scramble the eggs and milk together and pour over the vegetable mixture; then cook thoroughly. This is also excellent with 2 eggs (1 egg per person) *and* the tofu crumbled in.

Wild Blueberry Hot Breakfast

Serves: 2

> 2 cups frozen wild blueberries
> ½ cup soy, hemp, or almond milk
> ¼ cup unsweetened shredded coconut, lightly toasted
> ¼ cup chopped walnuts
> ¼ cup currants
> 1 banana, sliced

Heat frozen blueberries and soy milk until warm. Add remaining ingredients and stir well.

SMOOTHIES, BLENDED SALADS, AND OTHER DRINKS

Almond Hemp Nutri-Milk

Serves: 4

    1 cup hemp seeds
    1 cup raw almonds, soaked 6–8 hours
    2 Medjool dates (or 4 Deglet Noor), pitted
    2½ cups water
    ½ teaspoon vanilla

Place all ingredients in a Vitamix or other high-powered blender. Blend until smooth. Squeeze or strain through a cheesecloth, nut milk bag, or fine mesh strainer. Store in a glass jar.

To make chocolate Nutri-Milk, add 2–3 tablespoons natural cocoa powder to the blender along with other ingredients.

Cinnamon Apple Omega Milk

Serves: 4

    1 cup walnuts, soaked 6–8 hours
    1 cup raw cashews, soaked 6–8 hours
    ½ cup hemp seeds
    1 cup dried apple, soaked in 1 cup water until soft (save soak water)
    2 cups water
    1 teaspoon cinnamon

Place all ingredients in a Vitamix or other high-powered blender. Blend until smooth. Strain and squeeze through a cheesecloth, nut milk bag, or fine mesh strainer. Store in a glass jar.

Detox Green Tea

Serves: 4

    1 bunch kale
    2 cups romaine lettuce leaves
    1 cucumber
    4 leaves bok choy
    2 cups unsweetened green tea
    2 cups frozen raspberries
    2 cups frozen cherries or strawberries

Prepare a green juice by running the kale, romaine lettuce, cucumber, and bok choy through a juicer. Mix the green tea with 2 cups of the green juice. Add to a blender along with frozen raspberries and frozen cherries or strawberries and process until well blended.

Got Greens Smoothie

Serves: 2

    2 ounces fresh baby spinach
    2 ounces Boston or green leaf lettuce
    2 cups fresh or frozen pineapple cubes
    3 kiwis
    ½ avocado
    1 banana

Blend all ingredients in a Vitamix or other high-powered blender until smooth and creamy.

Purple Power Smoothie
Serves: 2

1 cup pomegranate juice
1 cup compacted baby spinach
1 cup compacted Boston lettuce
¼ medium cucumber
½ cup frozen blueberries
1 cup frozen mixed berries or strawberries
3 pitted dates
2 tablespoons ground flax seeds
1 cup ice

Blend ingredients in a Vitamix or other high-powered blender until smooth and creamy.

Very Berry Smoothie
Serves: 2

1 cup unsweetened soy, hemp, or almond milk
2 bananas
2 cups frozen peaches
½ cup frozen blackberries
½ cup frozen raspberries
½ cup frozen blueberries

Blend all ingredients in a Vitamix or other high-powered blender until smooth.

Waldorf Blended Salad
Serves: 1

½ cup pomegranate juice
1 apple, peeled and cored
¼ cup walnuts
3 cups compacted collard greens or kale
1 cup compacted lettuce
¼ cup water or ice cubes

Blend all ingredients in a Vitamix or other high-powered blender until smooth.

SALAD DRESSINGS

Banana Ginger Dressing
Serves: 2

    1 large banana
    ¼ cup fresh cilantro
    1 lemon, juiced
    1 tablespoon fresh ginger, chopped
    ½ teaspoon jalapeño pepper, seeded and chopped, or more to taste
    ¼ cup water

Blend all ingredients in a food processor or high-powered blender.

Goji Balsamic Dressing
Serves: 4

    ½ cup dried goji berries, soaked in ½ cup water to soften (reserve soaking water to use in recipe)
    2 teaspoons low-sodium mustard
    ¼ cup balsamic vinegar
    ¼ cup walnuts
    1 tablespoon minced scallions
    ½ teaspoon onion powder
    ½ cup no-salt-added or low-sodium vegetable broth
    Pinch black pepper

Place all ingredients in a high-powered blender. Blend until smooth.

Orange Cashame Dressing

Serves: 2

> ¼ cup unhulled sesame seeds
> ¼ cup raw cashews or ⅛ cup raw cashew butter
> ½ cup orange juice
> 2 tablespoons Dr. Fuhrman's Blood Orange Vinegar or Dr.
>   Fuhrman's Riesling Raisin Vinegar or 1 tablespoon rice vinegar
> 2 oranges, peeled, divided into segments, and cut into bite-size
>   pieces

Toast the sesame seeds in a dry skillet over medium-high heat for 3 minutes, shaking the pan almost continuously. In a blender or Vitamix, combine half the sesame seeds with all the cashews, orange juice, and vinegar. Add the orange pieces to the salad and mix in the blended dressing. Sprinkle the remaining sesame seeds on top. This tastes great on a spinach and mushroom salad with thinly sliced red onions, or a lettuce, tomato, and cucumber salad.

Peanut Ginger Dressing

Serves: 4

> 2 oranges, peeled and seeded
> ¼ cup rice vinegar
> ⅛ cup no-salt-added peanut butter
> ⅛ cup raw cashew butter or almond butter
> 1 teaspoon Bragg Liquid Aminos or low-sodium soy sauce
> ¼-inch piece fresh ginger, peeled
> ¼ clove garlic

Blend all ingredients in a high-powered blender until smooth.

Caesar's Secret Salad

Serves: 4

For the Salad:
½ cup raw almonds
2 tablespoons nutritional yeast
12 ounces romaine lettuce, chopped

For the Dressing:
6 cloves roasted garlic*
1 cup unsweetened soy, hemp, or almond milk
½ cup raw cashew butter
2 tablespoons nutritional yeast
2 tablespoons fresh lemon juice
1 tablespoon Dijon mustard
⅛ teaspoon black pepper

Blend almonds and the first 2 tablespoons of nutritional yeast together in a high-powered blender to form a "Parmesan" topping. Sprinkle over romaine lettuce. Blend all dressing ingredients together and pour over salad.

*To roast garlic, break the cloves apart, but leave the papery skins on. Roast at 350°F for about 15 minutes, until garlic becomes mushy. When cool, remove skins.

Marinated Kale Salad

Serves: 4

6 cups shredded kale
¼ cup currants
2 tablespoons goji berries
⅓ cup unsulfured, unsalted sun-dried tomatoes, finely chopped
½ cup sliced scallions
1 tablespoon fresh lemon juice
2 oranges, juiced
2 tablespoons pine nuts

Combine all ingredients except pine nuts in a mixing bowl. Mix the salad and crush the kale with your hands. Place the salad in a covered container in the refrigerator and let sit overnight. Toss before serving.

Nutri-Green Salad with Black Fig Dressing

Serves: 4

For the Salad:
>   3 ounces mâche*
>   3 ounces watercress
>   2 ounces frisée
>   4 ounces mixed baby greens
>   1 cup broccoli sprouts

For the Dressing:
>   ⅓ cup Dr. Fuhrman's Black Fig Vinegar or balsamic vinegar
>   1 teaspoon Dr. Fuhrman's VegiZest or other no-salt seasoning mix, adjusted to taste
>   4 tablespoons water
>   1 tablespoon Dijon mustard
>   1 teaspoon dried marjoram
>   1 tablespoon raw almond butter
>   1 tablespoon low-sodium ketchup
>   1 teaspoon garlic powder
>   ½ cup pecans, coarsely chopped

Wash and dry the salad ingredients and place in a large salad bowl. Whisk dressing ingredients, except for the pecans, until smooth. Toss salad with dressing; serve on plates topped with chopped pecans.

*Mâche is a mild salad lettuce with round small leaves. Use additional baby greens if mâche is not available.

Powerhouse Micro Salad

Serves: 1

    2 medium carrots, peeled
    ¼ small head cabbage
    1 cup broccoli pieces
    2 medium stalks celery
    1 large apple, cored
    ¼ cup pecans or other raw nuts
    1 teaspoon ground flax seeds

Using the S blade of a food processor, process ingredients until finely chopped, approximately the size of confetti. Pulse (turn on and off) several times during chopping. These ingredients store well, so the recipe can be increased to provide several servings.

Rainbow Chopped Salad

Serves: 4

    6 cups shredded bok choy
    2 cups carrots, cut in matchstick-size pieces
    1 cup finely shredded red cabbage
    ⅔ cup goji berries
    ⅔ cup slivered raw almonds
    1½ cups diced mango
    ¼ cup brown rice vinegar

Place all ingredients in a mixing bowl and mix well with your hands to rub the vinegar into the vegetables. Let the salad marinate for several hours before serving.

Variation: Pour leftover hot soup or sauce on top.

Spinach Salad with Strawberry Sesame Vinaigrette
Serves: 4

For the Salad:
> ½ cup raw whole pecans
> 12 ounces baby spinach
> 1 pint fresh strawberries, halved

For the Dressing:
> 2 cups fresh strawberries
> 4 pitted dates
> 1 tablespoon unhulled sesame seeds
> 3 tablespoons balsamic vinegar

Lightly toast pecans in a 250°F oven for 3 minutes and add them to the other salad ingredients in a bowl. Blend dressing ingredients in a high-powered blender until smooth. Pour over salad.

Triple Treat Cabbage Salad

Serves: 4

For the Salad:
  2 cups green cabbage, grated
  1 cup red cabbage, grated
  1 cup savoy cabbage, grated
  1 carrot, peeled and grated
  1 red pepper, thinly sliced
  4 tablespoons currants
  2 tablespoons raw pumpkin seeds
  2 tablespoons raw sunflower seeds
  1 tablespoon unhulled sesame seeds

For the Dressing:
  ⅓ cup unsweetened soy, hemp, or almond milk
  1 apple, peeled, cored, and sliced
  ½ cup raw cashews or ¼ cup raw cashew butter
  1 tablespoon Dr. Fuhrman's Spicy Pecan Vinegar or balsamic
    vinegar
  1 tablespoon currants, for garnish
  2 tablespoon unhulled sesame seeds, to be toasted for garnish

Lightly toast 2 tablespoons of the sesame seeds in a dry pan over
medium heat for 3 minutes, shaking the pan frequently. Mix all salad
ingredients together in a bowl. In a high-powered blender, blend soy
milk, apple, cashews, and vinegar; then toss with salad. Garnish with
dressing-portion currants and lightly toasted sesame seeds. This is
good made a day ahead to allow flavors to mingle.

Tropical Fruit Salad

Serves: 4

> 2 cups cubed pineapple
> 1 cup cubed mango
> 1 cup cubed papaya
> 2 oranges, peeled and sectioned
> 1 banana, sliced
> 2 tablespoons unsweetened shredded coconut
> Shredded romaine lettuce

Toss fruit together. Add coconut and serve on top of lettuce.

DIPS, SNACKS, AND CONDIMENTS

Black Bean and Corn Salsa

Serves: 8

> 1½ cups cooked black beans or 1 (15-ounce) can no-salt-added or
> low-sodium black beans, drained
> 1½ cups frozen white corn, thawed
> 4 medium fresh tomatoes, finely chopped
> ½ medium green bell pepper, finely chopped
> 1 small onion, finely chopped
> 3 large garlic cloves, finely chopped
> 2 jalapeño peppers (or more, if you like a hotter salsa), seeded
> and finely chopped
> ⅓ cup fresh cilantro, finely chopped
> 1½ tablespoons fresh lime juice
> 1½ tablespoons fresh lemon juice
> 1 tablespoon Dr. Fuhrman's VegiZest or other no-salt seasoning
> mix, adjusted to taste
> 1 teaspoon garlic powder, or to taste
> 1 teaspoon Bragg Liquid Aminos

Combine beans and corn in a mixing bowl. Add fresh tomatoes, pepper, onion, garlic, and jalapeños to bean and corn mixture along with remaining ingredients and mix thoroughly. Serve with raw vegetables or healthy tortilla chips.

To make healthy tortilla chips, cut sprouted-grain tortillas (such as Ezekiel's) into chip-size triangles, place on baking sheet, and bake at 200°F for 1 hour, or until crispy but not browned.

Note: Chopping can be done by food processor or by hand.

Eggplant Hummus
Serves: 4

1 medium eggplant, cut in half
1 cup cooked garbanzo beans (chickpeas) or 1 cup unsalted
   canned garbanzo beans, drained
⅓ cup water
4 tablespoons raw unhulled sesame seeds
2 tablespoons fresh lemon juice
1 tablespoon dried minced onions
4 cloves garlic, finely chopped
Dash paprika and/or dried parsley, for garnish

Bake eggplant at 350°F for 45 minutes. Let cool; remove skin and discard. Blend all ingredients, including baked, peeled eggplant, in a food processor or high-powered blender until smooth and creamy. Serve with assorted raw vegetables.

Golden Onion Morsels
Makes: 30–40 balls

1½ cups raw cashews
1 cup raw almonds
1 medium Golden Delicious apple, peeled, cored, and sliced
1 tablespoon nutritional yeast
1 teaspoon ground chia seeds
1 tablespoon onion powder
Toasted sesame seeds (for coating)
Minced chives (for coating)

Grind the cashews and almonds into a powdered meal in a high-powered blender; then add the apple slices, nutritional yeast, ground chia seeds, and onion powder and blend again. Form into small balls and roll each ball in the sesame seeds and chives.

Home-Style Ketchup

5 Medjool dates, pitted
1 cup water
2 (6-ounce) cans no-salt-added or low-sodium tomato paste
¼ cup white vinegar
½ teaspoon onion powder
½ teaspoon garlic powder

Blend water and dates in blender until very smooth. Pour into saucepan with other ingredients; whisk together on medium-low heat until bubbly. Chill before serving.

Island Black Bean Dip

Serves: 4

1½ cups cooked black beans or 1 (15-ounce) can no-salt-added or low-sodium black beans, drained and rinsed
2 teaspoons low-sodium salsa
¼ cup scallions, minced
1½ tablespoons Dr. Fuhrman's Blood Orange Vinegar or other fruity vinegar
2 tablespoons Dr. Fuhrman's MatoZest or other no-salt seasoning mix containing dried tomatoes, adjusted to taste
2 tablespoons minced red onion
½ cup finely diced mango
¼ cup finely diced red bell pepper
1 tablespoon minced fresh cilantro, for garnish

Remove ¼ cup of the black beans and set aside. Place remaining beans in a blender or food processor. Add salsa, scallions, vinegar, and MatoZest. Puree until relatively smooth. Adjust seasonings to taste. Transfer to a bowl and add the reserved black beans, red onion, mango, and red bell pepper. Mix well and chill for 1 hour. Garnish with cilantro. Serve with raw vegetables. Makes 2½ cups.

Seasoned Kale Chips and Popcorn

4–5 leaves kale, tough stems and center ribs removed, leaves
  chopped
6 cups air-popped popcorn
Olive oil
Water
1 tablespoon nutritional yeast
1–2 teaspoons chili powder

Spread kale evenly on a baking sheet. Bake in a 200°F oven for 30 minutes, or until kale is crispy and dry. Remove from oven and, when cool, combine with the popcorn. Add equal parts olive oil and water to a small spray bottle and shake well. Spray to very lightly coat the popcorn and kale; then mix in nutritional yeast and chili powder.

Simple Guacamole

Serves: 4

2 ripe avocados, peeled and pitted
½ cup finely chopped onion
¼ cup minced fresh cilantro
2 tablespoons fresh lime juice
¼ teaspoon ground cumin
¼ teaspoon freshly ground black pepper

Using a fork, mash the avocados in a small bowl. Add the remaining ingredients and stir well. Cover and chill.

SOUPS

"Cheesy" Kale Soup
Serves: 4

½ cup yellow split peas
1 onion, chopped
1 cup mushrooms, sliced
2 cups carrot juice
1 (15-ounce) can no-salt-added or low-sodium tomato sauce
1½ pounds kale, tough stems and center ribs removed, leaves
    coarsely chopped
¼ cup cashew butter
1 tablespoon nutritional yeast

In a pressure cooker, cover yellow split peas with about 2½ cups water and cook on high pressure for 6–8 minutes. Add remaining ingredients except cashew butter and cook on high pressure for 1 minute more. Release pressure and blend soup with cashew butter. Sprinkle with nutritional yeast before serving.

To make without a pressure cooker: Precook the split peas until soft. Combine cooked split peas with all remaining ingredients except cashew butter. Bring to a boil, reduce heat, and simmer until kale is tender (about 15 minutes). Add water as needed to achieve desired consistency. Stir in cashew butter. Sprinkle with nutritional yeast before serving.

Creamy Butternut Squash Soup with Mushrooms
Serves: 4

2 cups water
2 cups unsweetened soy, hemp, or almond milk
1 (15-ounce) can no-salt-added or low-sodium vegetable broth
6 carrots, cut in large chunks
5 celery stalks, sliced in chunks
2 onions, cut in half
2 medium zucchini, cut in large pieces
2 butternut squash, peeled and cubed
3 tablespoons Dr. Fuhrman's VegiZest or other no-salt seasoning
   mix, adjusted to taste
¼ teaspoon nutmeg
1 teaspoon salt-free Spike or Mrs. Dash seasoning
¼ teaspoon ground cloves
10 ounces shiitake, cremini, and/or oyster mushrooms, cut in
   half

Place all ingredients except mushrooms in soup pot. Bring to a boil; then reduce heat and simmer for 30 minutes. Pour soup into a food processor or blender and blend until smooth. Return soup to pot, add mushrooms, and simmer for another 30 minutes, or until mushrooms are tender.

Dr. Fuhrman's Famous Anticancer Soup

Serves: 10

> 1 cup dried split peas and/or beans
> 4 cups water
> 6–10 medium zucchini
> 5 pounds carrots, juiced (or 5–6 cups juice, purchased)*
> 2 bunches celery, juiced (or 2 cups juice, purchased)*
> 2 tablespoons Dr. Fuhrman's VegiZest or other no-salt seasoning
>   mix, adjusted to taste
> 4 medium onions, chopped
> 3 leek stalks, split lengthwise and separated to wash well, then
>   coarsely chopped
> 2 bunches kale, collard greens, or other greens, tough stems and
>   center ribs removed, leaves chopped
> 1 cup raw cashews
> 2½ cups fresh mushrooms (shiitake, cremini, and/or white),
>   chopped

Place the beans and water in a very large pot over low heat. Bring to a boil; then reduce heat and simmer. Add the zucchini whole to the pot. Add the carrot juice, celery juice, and VegiZest.

Put the onions, leeks, and kale in a blender and blend with a little bit of the soup liquid. Pour this mixture into the soup pot. Remove the softened zucchini with tongs and blend them in the blender with the cashews until creamy. Pour this mixture back into the soup pot. Add the mushrooms and continue to simmer until the beans are soft—about 2 hours total cooking time.

*Freshly juiced organic carrots and celery will maximize the flavor of this soup.

Golden Austrian Cauliflower Cream Soup

Serves: 4

- 1 head cauliflower, cut into pieces
- 3 carrots, coarsely chopped
- 1 cup coarsely chopped celery
- 2 leeks, split lengthwise and separated to wash well, then coarsely chopped
- 2 cloves garlic, minced
- 2 tablespoons Dr. Fuhrman's VegiZest or other no-salt seasoning mix, adjusted to taste
- 2 cups carrot juice
- 4 cups water
- ½ teaspoon nutmeg
- 1 cup raw cashews or ½ cup raw cashew butter
- 5 cups chopped kale leaves or baby spinach

Place all the ingredients except the kale (or spinach) and cashews in a pot and simmer for 15 minutes. In a food processor or high-powered blender, blend two-thirds of the ingredients with the cashews until smooth and creamy. Return to the pot and continue cooking for 10 minutes with the kale or spinach added.

Shiitake Watercress Soup

Serves: 4

2 large leeks, white and pale-green parts only, split lengthwise
and separated to wash well and cut into ½-inch slices

3 medium carrots, peeled and chopped

3 cloves garlic, chopped

3 cups shiitake mushrooms, sliced

6 cups no-salt-added or low-sodium vegetable broth

3 cups cooked white beans or 2 (15-ounce) cans low-sodium or
no-salt-added white beans, drained

5 cups watercress, tough stems removed

1 teaspoon herbes de Provence

Black pepper, to taste

Heat ⅛ cup water in a soup pot. Add leeks, carrot, and garlic and
water-sauté until tender, about 3 minutes. Add mushrooms and
cook an additional 3 minutes, or until mushroom juices are released.
Add vegetable broth, beans, watercress, and herbes de Provence and
simmer for 15 minutes. Ladle half the soup into a food processor or
high-powered blender and puree until smooth. Return soup to pot.

Nonvegan option: 4 ounces wild meat or fowl can be added to the soup
and then pulled out when cooked, to be shredded or chopped and
stirred back into soup.

Tomato Bisque
Serves: 4

3 cups carrot juice

1½ pounds chopped fresh tomatoes or 1 (28-oz) can no-salt-added or low-sodium whole tomatoes (San Marzano variety, if possible)

¼ cup sun-dried tomatoes, chopped

2 celery stalks, chopped

1 small onion, chopped

1 leek, split lengthwise and separated to wash well, chopped

1 large shallot, chopped

3 cloves garlic, chopped

2 tablespoons Dr. Fuhrman's MatoZest or other no-salt seasoning mix with dried tomatoes, adjusted to taste

1 teaspoon dried thyme, crumbled

1 small bay leaf

½ cup raw cashews or ¼ cup raw cashew butter

¼ cup chopped fresh basil

5 ounces baby spinach

In a large saucepan, add all ingredients except the cashews, basil, and spinach. Simmer for 30 minutes. Discard the bay leaf. Remove 2 cups of the vegetables with a slotted spoon and set aside. Puree the remaining soup with the cashews in a food processor or high-powered blender until smooth. Return the pureed soup along with the reserved vegetables to the pot. Stir in the basil and spinach and continue simmering for another few minutes, until spinach is wilted.

MAIN DISHES

Acorn Squash Supreme

Serves: 2

    1 large acorn squash
    4 tablespoons diced dried, unsulfured apricots, soaked until soft
    1½ cups pineapple, chopped
    2 tablespoons raisins
    2 tablespoons chopped raw cashews
    Cinnamon

Cut squash in half; after removing seeds, set the two pieces cut side down on a baking pan containing ½ inch water; bake for 30 minutes at 350°F.

Meanwhile, combine the apricots, pineapple, raisins, and cashews. After the squash has cooked, turn the pieces cut side up and scoop the fruit/nut mixture into the center of each piece. Return the squash to the pan and cover loosely with aluminum foil. Bake for an additional 30 minutes. Sprinkle with cinnamon; then put it back in the oven for 5 more minutes.

All-American Spinach with Mushrooms

Serves: 4

    2 medium onions, chopped
    1 teaspoon olive oil
    1 teaspoon nutritional yeast
    6 tablespoons Dr. Fuhrman's VegiZest or other no-salt seasoning
       mix, adjusted to taste
    6 cups shiitake mushrooms, chopped
    20 ounces fresh spinach

Water-sauté onions in ⅓ cup water mixed with 1 teaspoon olive oil for 5 minutes. Add mushrooms, VegiZest, and nutritional yeast; cook, stirring for an additional 5 minutes, or until mushrooms are tender. Add spinach, mix, and cook for 2 minutes, and then cover; shut off heat and let soup sit for another 5 minutes to let spinach fully wilt.

Bean Enchiladas

Serves: 6

1 medium green bell pepper, seeded and chopped
½ cup sliced onion
1 cup no-salt-added or low-sodium tomato sauce, divided
2 cups cooked pinto or black beans or 1 (15-ounce) can no-salt-added or low-sodium pinto or black beans, drained
1 cup frozen corn kernels
1 tablespoon chili powder
1 teaspoon ground cumin
1 teaspoon onion powder
⅛ teaspoon cayenne pepper, optional
1 tablespoon chopped fresh cilantro
6 corn tortillas

Sauté the green pepper and onion in 2 tablespoons of the tomato sauce until tender. Stir in the remaining tomato sauce, beans, corn, chili powder, cumin, onion powder, cilantro, and cayenne (if using). Spoon about ¼ cup of the bean mixture on each tortilla and roll up. Serve as is or bake for 15 minutes in a 375°F oven.

Better Burgers

Serves: 8

  1½ cups old-fashioned rolled oats (not quick or instant)
  1 cup ground walnuts
  1 cup water
  ¼ cup no-salt-added or low-sodium tomato paste
  ¼ cup Dr. Fuhrman's MatoZest or other no-salt seasoning mix
    containing dried tomatoes, adjusted to taste
  1 cup diced onion
  3 cloves garlic, minced
  6 cups finely minced mushrooms
  2 teaspoons dried basil
  ½ teaspoon dried oregano
  2 tablespoons fresh parsley, minced
  ⅔ cup frozen chopped spinach, thawed
  Freshly ground pepper, to taste

Preheat oven to 350°F. In a small saucepan, whisk together water, tomato paste, and MatoZest. Heat over medium-high heat until boiling. Shut off heat or flame and add rolled oats and ground walnuts. Stir well and set aside.

Water-sauté onion and garlic in a pan until onion is translucent. Then add mushrooms and additional water if needed. Cover and cook for 5 minutes more, or until mushrooms are tender.

In a large bowl, combine sautéed onions and mushrooms, oat/walnut mixture, spinach, and spices. Stir well to combine. With wet hands, shape mixture into 16 well-formed burgers and bake for 15 minutes on a lightly oiled baking sheet. Turn burgers to bake the other side for another 15 minutes. Serve on small whole-grain hamburger buns or whole-grain pita bread halves. Top with thinly sliced raw red onion and no-salt-added or low-sodium ketchup and shredded lettuce.

Nonvegan option: 8 ounces chopped white turkey meat can be added to the bowl and mixed in well before patties are formed, for a unique flavor.

Black Bean Lettuce Bundles

Serves: 4

 2 cups cooked black beans or 1 (15-ounce) can no-salt-added or
 low-sodium black beans, drained
 ½ large ripe avocado, peeled and pitted
 ½ medium green bell pepper, seeded and chopped
 3 green onions, chopped
 ⅓ cup chopped fresh cilantro
 ⅓ cup no-salt-added or low-sodium mild salsa
 2 tablespoons fresh lime juice
 1 clove garlic, minced
 1 teaspoon ground cumin
 8 large romaine lettuce leaves

In a bowl, mash the beans and avocado together with a fork until well
blended and only slightly chunky. Add all the remaining ingredients
except the lettuce, and mix.

Place approximately ¼ cup of the mixture in the center of each
lettuce leaf and roll up like a burrito.

Braised Kale and Squash with Pumpkin Seeds

Serves: 6

2 bunches kale, tough stems and center ribs removed, leaves
chopped

1 medium butternut squash or small pumpkin, peeled, seeded,
and cubed

2 medium red onions, coarsely chopped

6 cloves garlic, sliced

2 tablespoons Dr. Fuhrman's VegiZest or other no-salt seasoning
mix, adjusted to taste

⅔ cup water

3 tablespoons Dr. Fuhrman's Black Fig Vinegar or balsamic
vinegar

1 cup raw pumpkin seeds or sunflower seeds, lightly toasted*

Place kale, squash, onion, garlic, and VegiZest in a large pot with
water. Cover and steam over low heat for 20 minutes, or until kale
and squash are tender. Add vinegar and toss. Serve sprinkled with
lightly toasted pumpkin or sunflower seeds.

*Toast seeds in oven at 300°F for 4 minutes, or until lightly toasted.

Brussels Sprouts Polonaise

Serves: 3

6 cups brussels sprouts

¼ cup soft tofu

2 tablespoons lemon juice

2 dates, pitted

1 clove garlic, minced

1 tablespoon Dr. Fuhrman's VegiZest or other no-salt seasoning
mix, adjusted to taste

½ cup chopped fresh parsley, divided

½ cup unsweetened soy, hemp, or almond milk

Cut large sprouts in half; leave others intact. Steam for 8 minutes, or
until tender. Blend tofu, lemon juice, dates, garlic, VegiZest, ¼ cup
parsley, and soy milk in blender; then pour over sprouts. Sprinkle
with remaining parsley.

Creamy Cruciferous Curry
Serves: 4

2 onions, finely diced
4 cloves garlic, minced
3 carrots, diced
3 parsnips, diced
2 cups unsweetened soy, hemp, or almond milk
1 head cauliflower cut into small florets
2 cups sliced mushrooms
1 tablespoon curry powder
1 teaspoon turmeric
1 teaspoon cumin
2 cups cooked chickpeas or 1 (15-ounce) can no-salt-added or
  low-sodium chickpeas, drained
1 pound kale, tough stems removed, leaves chopped
1 cup frozen green peas
½ cup raw cashews, chopped

In a large pot over medium heat, water-sauté onions, garlic, carrots, and parsnips until onions are translucent (about 5 minutes). Stir in soy milk, cauliflower, mushrooms, curry powder, turmeric, and cumin and cook for 10 minutes, covered, over medium-low heat. Stir in kale, green peas, and chickpeas and continue to cook, covered, for another 15 minutes, or until vegetables are tender. Top each serving with chopped cashews.

Nonvegan option: 6 ounces diced chicken or turkey may be added to the first stage of the recipe.

Cremini Ratatouille

Serves: 2

    1 medium onion, thinly sliced
    2 garlic cloves, chopped
    2 large tomatoes, chopped, or 1 (15-ounce) can no-salt-added
       diced tomatoes
    1 medium eggplant, cut into 1-inch dice
    1 medium zucchini, sliced crosswise into 1-inch pieces
    10 ounces cremini or other mushrooms, sliced
    1 medium red pepper, cut into 1-inch pieces
    1 teaspoon oregano
    1 teaspoon basil
    Pepper to taste

Heat ⅛ cup water in a large, deep skillet. Water-sauté the onion until softened, about 3 minutes. Add the garlic and cook for 1 minute more, adding additional water as necessary to keep from scorching. Reduce the heat to moderately low and add the tomatoes, eggplant, zucchini, mushrooms, red pepper, and spices. Cover and cook, stirring occasionally, until vegetables are very tender, about 1 hour. Serve hot.

Easy Vegetable Pizza

Serves: 4

    4 large whole-grain pitas
    2 cups no-salt-added or low-sodium pasta sauce
    ½ cup chopped shiitake mushrooms
    ½ cup chopped red onion
    10 ounces frozen broccoli florets, thawed and finely chopped
    ½ cup shredded vegan mozzarella-type cheese alternative

Preheat the oven to 200°F. Place pitas on two baking sheets and warm for 10 minutes. Remove from oven and spoon on the pasta sauce. Sprinkle evenly with the mushrooms, onion, and broccoli. Add a light sprinkle of "cheese." Bake for 30 minutes.

Nonvegan option: You can use fresh mozzarella instead of the vegan cheese alternative, but in that case use a smaller amount; you can also use a mixture of vegan "cheese" and mozzarella.

Goji Chili Stew

Serves: 6

> 3 cups diced plum tomatoes or 1 (28-ounce) can no-salt-added or low-sodium plum tomatoes
> 1 pound frozen broccoli, thawed and chopped
> 10 ounces frozen chopped onions, thawed
> 2½ cups corn, fresh or frozen
> ½ cup goji berries
> 2 large zucchini, diced
> 4 ounces chopped mild green chilies
> 4 teaspoons chili powder, or more to taste
> 2 teaspoons cumin
> 3 cloves garlic, minced
> 1½ cups cooked pinto beans or 1 (15-ounce) can no-salt-added or low-sodium pinto beans, drained
> 1½ cups cooked black beans or 1 (15-ounce) can no-salt-added or low-sodium black beans, drained
> 1½ cups cooked red beans or 1 (15-ounce) no-salt-added or low-sodium red beans, drained

Cover and simmer all ingredients, except precooked (or canned) beans, for 20 minutes. Add beans and heat through.

Green Leafy Moroccan Medley
Serves: 4

1 tablespoon minced garlic
1½ cups diced onions
2 cups sliced mushrooms
1 red bell pepper, seeded and chopped
1 tablespoon ground coriander
1 tablespoon cinnamon
1 tablespoon ground cumin
1 teaspoon crushed red pepper
2 cups fire roasted tomatoes, no-salt-added or low-sodium
4 cups mustard greens, tough stems removed, leaves chopped
4 cups collard greens, tough stems removed, leaves chopped
¼ cup currants

In a large soup pot, heat 2 tablespoons water over medium-high heat and add the garlic and onions. Cook and stir for 5 minutes. Add the mushrooms, pepper, spices, and a little more water if needed. Cook and stir for another 5 minutes. Add all the remaining ingredients and simmer, covered, on medium-low heat for 10 minutes, or until the greens are tender.

Lisa's Lovely Lentil Stew

Serves: 4

> 2 cups dried lentils
> 6 cups water
> ½ medium onion, finely chopped
> 1 teaspoon dried basil
> ⅛ teaspoon black pepper
> 3 large ripe tomatoes, chopped
> 1 celery stalk, finely chopped

Place the lentils, water, onion, pepper, and basil in a pot and simmer for 30 minutes. Add the tomato and celery and simmer for an additional 15 minutes, or until lentils are tender.

Mighty Mushroom Stroganoff

Serves: 4

    2 onions, diced

    1 tablespoon minced garlic

    4 cups mushrooms

    2 teaspoons poultry seasoning

    2 cups dried mushrooms, such as shiitake and/or portobello, soaked in 2 cups water (keep the soak water)

    ½ cup cooking sherry or mirin rice wine

    1 tablespoon Dr. Fuhrman's VegiZest or other no-salt seasoning mix, adjusted to taste

    1½ cups frozen green peas

    8 cups chopped arugula

    8 ounces whole-wheat spiral pasta

For the Sauce:

    1 large head cauliflower, cored and broken into florets

    4 cups unsweetened soy, hemp, or almond milk

    2 cups cooked white beans or 1 (15-ounce) can no-salt-added or low-sodium white beans

    1 tablespoon tahini or unhulled sesame seeds

    1 teaspoon Mrs. Dash no-salt seasoning

    1 tablespoon onion powder

    1 tablespoon nutritional yeast

In a soup pot, sauté the onion and garlic in a little water for 5 minutes. Add the fresh mushrooms and the poultry seasoning and sauté for another 5 minutes. Add the dried mushrooms with their soaking water. Cook and stir until the mushrooms are soft. Add the cooking sherry, peas, and arugula and cook for another 10 minutes.

To prepare the sauce, place the cauliflower and soy milk in a saucepan and bring to a boil uncovered. Reduce the heat and let simmer on low, covered for 15 minutes, or until cauliflower is fork-tender. Add the remaining ingredients and puree in a blender until smooth. Add the cauliflower sauce to the mushroom mixture and stir well.

Meanwhile, cook pasta according to package directions. Drain and reserve 1 cup of the cooking water. Combine pasta with cauliflower sauce and mushroom mixture, adding reserved cooking water to moisten if necessary.

Nonvegan option: 5–6 ounces grass-fed or wild meat, cubed, can be added to the sauté pot with the mushrooms, for a more traditional Hungarian flavor.

Portobello Mushrooms and Beans

Serves: 4

1 large onion, chopped
2 garlic cloves, chopped
2 large portobello mushroom caps, sliced thin
½ cup red wine or low-sodium vegetable broth
1 large tomato, diced, or 8 halved cherry tomatoes
1½ cups cooked garbanzo beans or 1 (15-ounce) can no-salt-added or low-sodium garbanzo beans, drained

Water-sauté the onion and garlic for 2 minutes, or until onion is soft. Add the mushrooms and the red wine or broth and continue cooking for 5 minutes, until mushrooms are tender. Add the tomatoes and garbanzo beans. Simmer for 5 minutes.

Spaghetti Squash Primavera

Serves: 4

1 medium spaghetti squash
1½ carrots, diagonally sliced
½ cup celery, diagonally sliced
3 cloves garlic, minced
1½ cups shredded cabbage
1 small zucchini, chopped into small pieces
1½ cups cooked pinto beans or 1 (15-ounce) can no-salt-added or
    low-sodium pinto beans, drained
1½ cups chopped tomatoes or 1 (15-ounce) can no-salt-added or
    low-sodium chopped tomatoes, drained
⅓ cup apple juice
1 teaspoon dried thyme
1 teaspoon dried parsley
1 cup no-salt-added or low-sodium pasta sauce
1 head romaine lettuce leaves (optional), shredded

Slice spaghetti squash in half lengthwise; remove seeds. Place both
halves cut side down on a baking pan containing ¼ cup water. Bake
for 45 minutes at 350°F, or until tender.

Meanwhile, cook carrots and celery in 2 tablespoons water in a
covered pan over medium heat for 10 minutes, stirring occasionally.
Add a little more water if needed. Add garlic, cabbage, and zucchini
and cook, covered, for another 10 minutes. Stir in remaining
ingredients, except for pasta sauce. Cover and simmer for 10 minutes,
or until carrots are tender.

When squash is done, remove from oven and use a fork to scrape
spaghetti-like strands from squash into a bowl. Add pasta sauce and
combine by mixing thoroughly. Mix the vegetables, beans, and herbs
with the squash/pasta sauce mixture and serve on a bed of shredded
romaine lettuce (if desired) or place back in the hollowed-out squash
bowls.

Super Food Stuffed Peppers

Serves: 3

½ cup dry quinoa

3 large bell peppers, cut in half lengthwise, seeds and membranes
   removed

3 cloves garlic, minced

1 medium onion, minced

1 medium eggplant, diced

1 medium zucchini, diced

8 ounces mushrooms, diced

1½ cups no-salt-added or low-sodium tomato sauce or 1
   (15-ounce) can crushed or diced no-salt-added or low-sodium
   tomatoes

1 teaspoon dried oregano or Italian seasoning (or more to taste)

2 tablespoons fresh basil, optional

Add quinoa to 1¼ cups water in a covered pot and simmer on low
heat for 20 minutes. Water-sauté the garlic and onion. Add the
eggplant, zucchini, and mushrooms and cook until eggplant and
zucchini start to soften. Add the cooked quinoa, tomato sauce or
crushed tomatoes, and seasonings. Spoon vegetable/quinoa mixture
into peppers and bake for 15 minutes at 350°F.

Swiss Chard and Sweet Potato Gratin
Serves: 6

1 teaspoon chopped fresh ginger
1 small onion, finely chopped
½ cup chopped pepper
8 cups Swiss chard, stems removed, coarsely chopped
4 medium (about 1¼ pounds) sweet potatoes, peeled, sliced
⅛ inch thick
8 ounces tempeh, sliced as thinly as possible
2 cups unsweetened hemp, soy, or almond milk
⅛ teaspoon nutmeg
⅛ teaspoon black pepper
¼ cup nondairy mozzarella "cheese"
2 tablespoons flax seeds, toasted

Preheat oven to 400°F. Rub a 9 x 13–inch baking dish with a small amount of olive oil. Heat ⅛ cup water in a large pan and water-sauté ginger, onion, and green pepper until softened. Add Swiss chard and cook until just tender. Arrange one-third of sliced sweet potatoes on bottom of prepared baking dish. Place half of tempeh and half of Swiss chard mixture on top. Arrange another one-third of sweet potato slices and remaining tempeh and Swiss chard, followed by remaining sweet potato. Combine milk, nutmeg, and black pepper. Pour over dish. Cover with foil and bake for 35 minutes. Remove foil, top with nondairy mozzarella "cheese," and bake for an additional 15 minutes. Sprinkle with toasted flax seeds.

Nonvegan option: Use a small amount of fresh mozzarella in place of the nondairy cheese alternative; it is a very small amount per person either way.

Tangy White Beans and Zucchini

Serves: 2

3 medium zucchini, cut into small chunks

2 cloves garlic, minced

1½ cups cooked white beans or 1 (15-ounce) can no-salt-added or low-sodium white beans, drained

¼ cup Dr. Fuhrman's Black Fig Vinegar or balsamic vinegar

Sauté zucchini and garlic in 2 tablespoons water over medium heat for 5 minutes or until tender. Add beans and vinegar and cook for 5 minutes.

Thai Longevity Stew

Serves: 4

6 cloves garlic, chopped
2 teaspoons minced ginger
1½ tablespoons minced jalapeño pepper
3 cups sliced leeks, split lengthwise and separated to wash well,
     then coarsely chopped
2 cups quartered mushrooms
1 cup shredded carrots
1 cup shredded cabbage
2 cups snow peas
½ cup unsalted, unsweetened peanut butter
1 cup no-salt-added or low-sodium vegetable broth
½ cup unsweetened soy, hemp, or almond milk
½ cup unsweetened shredded coconut
1 lime, juiced
Crushed red pepper or cayenne pepper, to taste
2 tablespoons chopped fresh cilantro, for garnish

In a large soup pot, heat 2 tablespoons water over medium-high heat
and add the garlic, ginger, jalapeño pepper, leeks, and mushrooms.
Cook and stir for 5 minutes. Add the carrots, cabbage, and snow
peas and a little more water if needed. Cook and stir for another 5
minutes, or until vegetables are tender.

In a small bowl, mix together the peanut butter with some of the
vegetable broth to make a smooth sauce. Add the peanut butter
mixture, the remaining broth, and the soy milk, coconut, and lime
juice to the stew. Add crushed red pepper or cayenne pepper if
desired. Serve hot, garnished with cilantro.

Nonvegan option: 6 ounces shrimp or scallops can be chopped and
added to the pot.

PITA/WRAP STUFFERS
Aztec Stuffer

Serves: 2

> 2 cups very finely shredded collard greens
> ¼ cup low-sodium salsa
> ¼ cup raw almond butter
> ¼ cup fresh cilantro, minced
> 1 teaspoon ground cumin
> 1 teaspoon chili powder

In a bowl, mix everything together. Serve stuffed into a whole-grain pita or wrap.

Italian Stuffer

Serves: 2

> 2 cups shredded lettuce
> ¼ cup chopped parsley
> ¼ cup chopped sun-dried tomatoes, unsalted, soaked until soft
> ½ cup finely ground walnuts
> 1 teaspoon no-salt Italian seasoning
> 1½ tablespoons no-salt-added or low-sodium tomato paste
> Pinch garlic powder

In a bowl, mix everything together. Serve stuffed into a whole-grain pita or wrap.

Nonvegan option: Add 1–2 ounces oven-baked white-meat chicken or turkey, sliced or chopped, to each wrap.

Mumbai Stuffer

Serves: 2

> 2 cups shredded green cabbage
> ¼ cup diced dried mango
> ¼ cup raw almond butter
> 1 teaspoon curry powder
> 2 tablespoons orange juice, freshly squeezed

In a bowl, mix everything together. Serve stuffed into a whole-grain pita or wrap.

DESSERTS

Apple Berrynut Bites

Serves: 12

2 cups dried apples
1½ cups unsweetened vanilla soy, hemp, or almond milk
1 pint fresh strawberries or 1 bag frozen
½ cup raw pecans
½ cup raw Brazil nuts
1 cup baby spinach
¼ cup unsweetened shredded coconut
½ tablespoon cinnamon
¼ teaspoon nutmeg
6 Medjool dates, pitted
Unsweetened shredded coconut, for garnish

Soak dried apples in soy milk for at least an hour. In a high-powered blender combine soaked apples, soy milk, and half the strawberries with remaining ingredients, except for coconut, until smooth. Add a little more soy milk if needed. Spoon into muffin cups or small oven-proof custard cups and bake for 20 minutes at 300°F. Using remaining strawberries, place half a berry on top of each pudding cup and sprinkle with coconut. Chill in refrigerator before serving.

Berry Boost Gelatin

Serves: 2

2 cups unsweetened apricot nectar
3 teaspoons agar flakes, soaked overnight in the apricot nectar
2 cups mixed fresh or frozen berries, chopped into small chunks
1 teaspoon vanilla extract

Place apricot nectar/agar flake mixture in a small saucepan. Bring to a boil over medium-high heat; then reduce heat to simmer and continue cooking for 20 minutes. Stir in the berries and vanilla. Divide into 2 serving dishes and chill before serving.

Black Bean Brownies

Makes: 16 squares

2 cups cooked black beans
10 Medjool dates or 5 date rolls
2½ tablespoons raw almond butter
1 teaspoon vanilla
½ cup natural, nonalkalized cocoa powder
1 tablespoon ground chia seeds

Combine the black beans, dates, almond butter, and vanilla in a food processor or high-powered blender. Blend until smooth. Add the remaining ingredients and blend again. Pour into a very lightly oiled 8 x 8–inch baking pan. Bake/dehydrate at 200°F for 1½ hours. Cool before cutting into small squares. Store in a covered container in the refrigerator for up to one week.

Black Cherry Sorbet

Serves: 3

3 cups frozen sweet black cherries
1 cup vanilla soy, hemp, or almond milk
1 frozen ripe banana*
½ cup walnuts
3 Medjool dates, pitted

Blend all the ingredients in a high-powered blender and serve.

*Freeze peeled ripe banana in a plastic bag at least 24 hours in advance.

Chia Cookies
Makes: 20 cookies

    2 cups finely ground rolled oats
    ½ cup dried, unsweetened shredded coconut
    1 cup currants
    1 tablespoon ground chia seeds
    1 tablespoon whole chia seeds
    1 teaspoon cinnamon
    2 tablespoons raw almond butter
    ¾ cup unsweetened applesauce
    1 teaspoon vanilla

Soak about half the currants in ½ cup water for 1 hour.

Combine the ground oats, coconut, remaining currants, chia seeds, and cinnamon in a bowl.

Preheat oven to 200°F. Place the almond butter, soaked currants and their soak water, applesauce, and vanilla in a food processor or high-powered blender. Blend until smooth, then add to the remaining ingredients and mix well.

Form cookies using 2 teaspoons of dough per cookie. Place on a baking sheet lightly wiped with oil or covered with parchment paper. Bake at very low heat, 200°F, for 1½ to 2 hours.

Chocolate Dip with Fresh Fruit and Berries
Serves: 4

    2 cups baby spinach
    1½ cups soy milk
    1 cup frozen blueberries
    1 cup pitted dates
    ⅔ cup raw almonds
    2½ tablespoons nonalkalized, unsweetened cocoa powder
    ½ teaspoon vanilla extract
    4 tablespoons goji berries

Place all the ingredients in a high-powered blender. Blend until very smooth and creamy.

Serve as a dip for fresh fruit, or spoon over sliced fruit and berries.

Chunky Blueberry Walnut Sorbet

Serves: 4

> 1 cup unsweetened soy, hemp, or almond milk
> 3 cups frozen blueberries, divided
> 2 frozen bananas,* one chopped into bite-size pieces
> 1 cup chopped walnuts, divided
> 1 tablespoon ground flax seeds

Blend soy milk, 2 cups frozen blueberries, 1 frozen banana (unchopped), and ½ cup walnuts in high-powered blender. Empty into a chilled bowl and mix in remaining blueberries and walnuts. Served topped with ground flax seeds.

*Freeze ripe bananas at least 24 hours in advance. To freeze, peel, cut into thirds, and wrap tightly in plastic.

Coconut Carrot Cream Pie

Serves: 8

For the Filling:
- ½ cup muscat or other sweet dessert wine
- 3 apples, grated
- 1 cup dried apples, unsulfured, chopped
- ⅓ cup raisins
- ⅓ cup dried apricots, unsulfured, chopped
- ¼ cup walnuts
- 1½ cups shredded carrots
- ½ cup shredded zucchini
- ½ cup shredded beets
- ½ cup unsweetened shredded coconut
- ¾ teaspoon cinnamon
- ¼ teaspoon nutmeg

For the Pie Crust:
- 1 cup raw almonds
- 1 cup dates, pitted
- 2 tablespoons chia seeds
- ⅓ cup dry oatmeal (ground in blender)

For the Icing:
- 1⅓ cup macadamia nuts
- 1 cup soy, hemp, or almond milk
- ⅔ cup pitted dates
- 1 teaspoon vanilla

For the filling, marinate chopped dried apples and apricots in wine overnight (or for at least 1 hour) in the refrigerator. Combine raisins and walnuts in a food processor or blender and add the fruit/wine mixture; process together until combined. Add coconut, cinnamon, and nutmeg, and hand-mix with the finely shredded (but not blended) carrots, zucchini, and beets.

For pie crust, mix 2 tablespoons chia seeds in ¼ cup water and let stand for at least 15 minutes. Combine in food processor into a paste; then set paste aside. Place almonds in food processor and process until very fine; set aside. Process the oatmeal into a coarse oat flour by blending dry; then return the almonds to the blender and mix with the oat flour. Add dates and process until chopped and mixed well with other ingredients. Add chia seed paste and pulse to mix in. Press mixture into a pie plate to form shell.

For the icing, blend macadamia nuts, soy milk, the second batch of dates, and vanilla until smooth and creamy in a high-powered blender.

Golden Delicious Truffles
Makes: 30–40 balls

> 1½ cups raw cashews
> 1 cup raw almonds
> 1 medium Golden Delicious apple, peeled, cored, and sliced
> 1 teaspoon ground chia seeds
> 8 dried apricots, minced
> Cinnamon (for coating)
> Unsweetened shredded coconut (for coating)
> Natural, nonalkalized cocoa powder (for coating)

Grind the cashews and almonds into a powdered meal in a Vitamix or other high-powered blender; then add the apple slices, ground chia seeds, and dried apricot, and blend again. To make truffles, form mixture into small balls and roll each ball in either the cinnamon or a mixture of coconut and cocoa powder.

Healthy Chocolate Cake

Serves: 12

For the Cake:

> 1⅔ cups whole-wheat flour
> 1 teaspoon baking powder
> 3 teaspoons baking soda
> 3½ cups pitted dates, divided
> 1 cup pineapple chunks in own juice, drained
> 1 banana
> 1 cup unsweetened applesauce
> 1 cup shredded raw beets
> ¾ cup shredded raw carrots
> ½ cup shredded raw zucchini
> 3 tablespoons natural, nonalkalized cocoa powder
> ½ cup currants
> 1 cup chopped walnuts
> 1½ cups water
> 2 teaspoons vanilla extract

For the Chocolate Nut Icing:

> 1 cup raw macadamia nuts and/or raw cashews
> 1 cup vanilla soy, hemp, or almond milk
> ⅔ cup pitted dates
> ⅓ cup brazil nuts or hazelnuts
> 2 tablespoons cocoa powder
> 1 teaspoon vanilla extract

Preheat oven to 350°F. Mix flour, baking powder, and baking soda in a small bowl. Set aside. In blender or food processor, puree 3 cups of the dates, pineapple, banana, and applesauce. Slice remaining ½ cup dates into ¼-inch pieces. In large bowl, mix sliced dates, beets, carrots, zucchini, cocoa powder, currants, walnuts, water, vanilla, and flour mixture. Add the blended mixture and mix well. Spread in a 9 x 13–inch nonstick baking pan.

Bake for 1 hour or until a toothpick inserted into the center comes out clean. For the icing, use a high-powered blender and combine all icing ingredients until smooth and creamy. Spread on cooled cake.

Wild Blueberry Apple Pie

Serves: 8

For the Crust:
> 1 cup raw almonds
> 1 teaspoon finely ground chia seeds
> 1 cup pitted dates
> 2 teaspoons water

For the Pie Filling:
> ½ cup water
> ½ cup pitted dates
> 1 apple, peeled, cored, and chopped
> 2 teaspoons finely ground chia seeds
> 1 cup frozen wild blueberries, slightly thawed
> 4 medium apples, peeled, cored, and sliced
> 1 tablespoon cinnamon
> ½ cup raisins

To make the crust, combine the raw almonds and the first batch of chia seed powder in a food processor. Pulse until finely ground. Add the dates and water and process until the mixture gathers into a ball. Press the mixture to form a thin crust in a very lightly oiled 8-inch pie plate. Prebake the crust for 5 minutes at 250°F.

To make the filling, combine the water, pitted dates, chopped apple, and second batch of chia seed powder in a blender. Blend until smooth. In a large mixing bowl, combine the date mixture with the blueberries, sliced apples, cinnamon, and raisins. Mix well. Spoon the filling into the pie crust and bake at 200°F for 1½ hours. Chill before slicing and serving.

Glossary

Acute illness: A disease with an abrupt onset and usually a short course.

Adenoma: A benign (noncancerous) tumor that develops from epithelial tissue. Adenomas can grow from many organs and, over time, may progress into a malignant (cancerous) tumor.

Amino acid: A class of molecules made of nitrogen, carbon, and oxygen. The building blocks of proteins, they are crucial to metabolism. Twenty amino acids exist in nature; the human body produces eleven of them; the other nine must be supplied by food.

Anemia: A condition in which the body does not have enough healthy red blood cells. Red blood cells provide oxygen to body tissues.

Angiogenesis: The new growth of blood vessels from preexisting blood vessels. This is a normal process in growth and development, as well as in wound healing; however, it is also a fundamental step in the transition of tumors from a harmless state to a malignant (cancerous) state.

Angiogenesis inhibitor: A substance that inhibits angiogenesis (the growth of blood vessels). Every solid tumor needs to generate the growth of new blood vessels to feed itself once it reaches a certain size. Thus an angiogenesis inhibitor acts, indirectly, to slow or prevent the growth of a tumor.

Antigen: Any substance that causes the immune system to produce antibodies against it. Antigens may be foreign substances from the environment (chemicals, bacteria, viruses, or pollens) or may be formed within the body.

Antimicrobial: A substance that inhibits growth of microorganisms. A class of drugs referred to as antimicrobials consists of antibiotics, antifungals, and antivirals.

Antioxidant: A substance that protects cells against the effects of damaging free radicals by neutralizing or stabilizing them. Antioxidants are found in fruits, vegetables, nuts, and grains.

Apoptosis: A process of cellular death in which a cell is signaled to undergo self-degradation. This is the body's way of disposing of damaged or unneeded cells.

Aromatase inhibitor: A substance or drug that inhibits or slows the production of the hormone estrogen. These drugs are often used in the treatment of estrogen-related cancers, such as breast and ovarian cancer.

Atherosclerosis: A condition in which fatty material collects along the walls of arteries, forming a thick and hardened plaque. This plaque reduces blood flow to the heart and may result in chest pain and cause heart attack or stroke.

Bacteremia: The presence of bacteria in the blood. This typically leads to septic shock and can be fatal.

B cells: Lymphocytes (white blood cells) that play a large role in immune system defense against microbes. The principal functions of B cells are to make antibodies against antigens, perform the role of antigen-presenting cells, and eventually develop into memory B cells after activation by antigen interaction. B cells are an essential component of the adaptive immune system.

Beriberi: A disease caused by the body's lack of thiamine (vitamin B_1). Beriberi can affect the cardiovascular system or the nervous system and is fatal if not treated. This disease can be prevented by a diet containing B_1, rich in vegetables, nuts, and whole grains.

Cancer cells: Cells that have lost their ability to divide in a *controlled* fashion, which leads to uncontrolled or rapid cell division and growth—that is, tumor development. A malignant (or cancerous) tumor consists of a population of rapidly dividing cancer cells that may eventually travel to other locations in the body.

Carcinogen: An agent that causes cancer. Commonly known carcinogens include asbestos, arsenic, and tobacco smoke. In food, carcinogens may be found in pesticides or in plastic packaging. Carcinogens can also be formed during the process of cooking foods at high temperatures, such as grilling, roasting, or frying.

Carotenoids: Naturally occurring chemicals with nutritive properties that exist in the pigment that colors fruits and vegetables. They act as antioxidants and can be converted into essential vitamins by the body.

Cervical dysplasia: Abnormal changes in the cells on the surface of the cervix, which is the lower part of the uterus (womb), where it opens at the top of the vagina. Although these cell changes are not cancer, they can lead to cancer of the cervix if not treated or removed.

Chronic illness: A disease characterized by a long duration and generally slow progression.

Coronary vessels: Blood vessels that supply the heart muscle with blood.

Cretinism: A condition, present from birth, caused by a deficiency of iodine or thyroid hormone during prenatal development. The condition is characterized by dwarfism and mental retardation.

Crohn's disease: A condition characterized by inflammation of the digestive tract. This disease causes abdominal pain or diarrhea, which can lead to malnutrition. The exact cause remains unknown, but is associated with a problem with the body's immune system.

Dendritic cells: A special type of cell that is a key regulator of the immune system. These cells trap foreign material, which is later destroyed by other immune cells.

Detoxification: The body's efforts to reduce its toxic load by changing irritants to a less harmful form, or one that can be more readily eliminated; or the body's efforts to force the expulsion of such substances through channels of elimination, such as mucus, urine, or skin.

DHA (docosahexaenoic acid): An omega-3 fatty acid important for normal brain function and the development of the nervous system. The body can manufacture DHA from alpha-linolenic acid, found in seeds and greens, or get it directly from certain fish, from an algae-derived supplement, or from a fish oil supplement.

Endogenous waste: A waste product that originates from within an organism, tissue, or cell.

Enzyme: A type of protein that increases the rate of a chemical reaction, without being destroyed or altered in the process.

EPA (eicosapentaenoic acid): An omega-3 fatty acid that has the ability to reduce inflammation, inhibit cancer development, and protect blood vessels. EPA can be obtained from fish, supplements of fish oils, or special yeast.

Epigenetic change: An intracellular change in gene activity and expression that does not involve alterations to the genetic code but still gets passed down to at least one successive generation. Genetic changes can result from environmental or external factors.

Exogenous waste: A noxious substance that originates outside of an organism, cell, or tissue.

Flavonoid: A polyphenolic compound that is ubiquitous in nature. Over 4,000 flavonoids have been identified in colorful fruits and vegetables and are known to have antiviral, anti-allergic, anti-inflammatory, antitumor, and antioxidant activities.

Flexitarian: A person who eats a mostly vegetarian, plant-based diet but will occasionally eat animal products such as meat, poultry, or fish.

Free radical: An atom or molecule with an odd number of electrons. The resulting "unpaired" electrons make the free radical reactive and unstable. Once formed, free radicals start a chain reaction that can damage important cellular components, such as DNA. Free-radical damage can result in a variety of diseases and even cancers.

Gene: A sequence of DNA that codes for specific proteins that determine an organism's characteristics. The information stored in genes is passed from generation to generation.

Glucosinolate: A class of protective phytochemicals that occur naturally in cruciferous vegetables (broccoli, cabbage, kale, cauliflower, etc.). Approximately 120 different glucosinolates help the body eliminate carcinogens and give cruciferous vegetables a mildly bitter taste.

Goiter: A condition resulting from a lack of iodine in the diet. Goiter causes the thyroid gland to enlarge, leading to a visible swelling at the front of the neck.

Homocysteine: An intermediate protein in the synthesis of the amino acid cysteine, which increases as a result of certain nutritional deficiencies (especially vitamin B_{12} or folate). The elevation of homocysteine has been implicated in coronary artery disease and heart attacks.

Immune memory: The immune system's ability to recognize and deal with a previously encountered pathogen. If the body is reinfected with a pathogen it has previously overcome, it will have an adapted subpopulation of B cells on hand to provide a very specific and rapid secondary response. This secondary response is usually so fast and efficient that we are not aware we have been reinfected.

Inoculum: The collection of microbes or viral load being introduced into the body.

Interferon: A protein made in the body in response to the presence of pathogens (viruses, bacteria, parasites) or cancerous cells. Interferons allow communication between cells and trigger the protective defenses of the immune system to kill invading pathogens.

Isothiocyanates (ITCs): Sulfur-containing phytochemicals formed from the glucosinolates present in cruciferous vegetables. ITCs neutralize carcinogens (cancer-causing substances), inhibit cellular proliferation or rapid growth, and induce cellular death.

Laryngeal Papillomas: Benign (noncancerous) epithelial tumors that affect the larynx and upper respiratory tract. They are caused by infection with the human papilloma virus (HPV).

Lymphocytes: The white blood cells primarily responsible for protection against viral illnesses. The three major types of lymphocyte are T cells, B cells, and natural killer (NK) cells.

Natural killer (NK) cells: A type of lymphocyte (white blood cell) and a component of the immune system. NK cells play a major role in defense against abnormal (dysplastic) cells that could develop into tumors and cancers, as well as virally infected cells. NK cells distinguish infected cells and tumors from normal and uninfected cells by recognizing level changes of a surface molecule called MHC (major histocompatibility complex). Activated NK cells release cytotoxic (cell-killing) granules, which then destroy the abnormal cells.

Natural killer T (NKT) cells: A subset or type of T cell that has natural killer (NK) cell molecular markers on its surface. Not to be confused with NK cells, NKT cells share properties of both T cells and NK cells. They produce interferon and other chemo-attractive molecules that activate an immune response.

Macronutrients: Fats, carbohydrates, and proteins, which supply calories (energy) and are necessary for growth and normal function.

Macrophage: A large scavenger cell that engulfs and destroys bacteria and other foreign debris. Macrophages are involved in the immune response and help destroy bacteria, protozoa, and tumor cells. They present antigens and release substances that stimulate other cells of the immune system, such as neutrophils and T cells, to join the attack. As scavengers, macrophages rid the body of worn-out cells and other debris.

Malignant: The tendency of a medical condition, especially a tumor, to become progressively worse. In routine use, the word refers to a tumor that is cancerous. A malignant tumor (cancer) is capable of spreading to nearby tissues.

Meningitis: A potentially dangerous infection that affects the brain and spinal cord. Bacterial meningitis is a more serious condition than viral meningitis.

Methylation: The addition of a simple four-atom molecule (one carbon and three hydrogen atoms, known as a "methyl group") to a substance. The addition or removal of a methyl group creates changes in the DNA and has been associated with the development of cancer.

Microbe or microorganism: A microscopic living organism, such as bacterium, fungus, protozoan, or virus. It is arguable whether a virus is living or not since it cannot reproduce outside a host, but it is still considered a microbe.

Micronutrients: Essential dietary elements required in small quantities for various bodily needs, but not a source of calories. Micronutrients include minerals, vitamins, and phytochemicals.

Mortality rate: A measure of the number of deaths in a population.

Mucilage: A thick, gluey substance produced by most plants.

Neutrophil: A type of white blood cell designed to fight off infections and diseases that enter the body. Neutrophils are filled with tiny sacs of enzymes that kill and digest microorganisms that the neutrophils surround and swallow. An increased amount of neutrophils in the blood is a common finding with bacterial infections. During the beginning phase of a bacterial infection, neutrophils are among the first responders, tackling inflammation in particular.

Nosocomial infection: An infection that occurs as a result of treatment in a hospital or health care facility.

Nutritarian: A person who has a preference for foods and/or a health-promoting diet-style high in micronutrients. This word was coined by Dr. Fuhrman.

Omega-3 fatty acid: A class of fatty acid that includes ALA (alpha-linolenic acid) from vegetables, seeds, and nuts, but also includes the longer-chain omega-3s, EPA and DHA, which are commonly found in fish oil (but which the body can manufacture from ALA). Omega-3 fatty acids confer a number of health benefits and are necessary for optimal functioning of the immune system, brain, and cardiovascular system.

Oncologist: A physician who studies, diagnoses, and treats cancer.

Osteoarthritis: A common joint disorder in which joints of the body are stiff or painful and difficult to move.

Osteoporosis: A common bone disease in which bones become thinner and less dense over time.

Otitis media: Commonly referred to as an ear infection, or inflammation of the middle ear.

Pathogen: An infection agent, such as a virus, bacterium, or fungus, that can cause disease.

Pellagra: A disease that occurs when a person does not get enough niacin (one of the B vitamins) or tryptophan (an amino acid). Pellagra can cause dementia, diarrhea, skin disease, and even death.

Phenol: Chemical compound found in plant products that acts as an antioxidant.

Phytochemicals: Numerous newly discovered micronutrients present in plant foods with substantial ability to maximize the body's defenses against developing disease, including protection from toxins and carcinogens.

Phytoestrogen: A group of chemicals found in beans, seeds, and grains that can act like the hormone estrogen.

Placebo: An inactive pill, medication, or treatment that is used in studies as a standard against which the active, experimental treatment is compared.

Prebiotics: Foods or supplements that promote the growth of probiotics.

Probiotics: Bacteria that help maintain the natural balance of beneficial organisms (microflora) in the intestines.

Rickets: A disorder caused by lack of vitamin D, calcium, or phosphate. Any of these deficiencies, but especially all in combination, lead to softening and weakening of the bones.

Scurvy: A disease caused by lack of vitamin C. Scurvy can cause general weakness, anemia, gum disease, and skin hemorrhages.

Standard American diet (SAD): A dietary habit chosen by many people in developed countries, especially America. It is characterized by high intakes of animal products, sweets, cooking oils, high-fat foods, and processed foods. SAD is associated with heart disease and cancers.

Streptococcus pneumoniae: A type of bacterium that causes pneumonia, otitis media (ear infection), and bacterial meningitis.

T cell or *T lymphocyte:* A type of white blood cells that plays a central role in cell-mediated immunity. The abbreviation T, in T cell, stands for "thymus," the principal organ responsible for the T cell's maturation. Several different subsets of T cells have been discovered, each with a distinct function. The types include memory T cells, responsible for immune memory to prior antigens and infections, and cytotoxic T cells for killing viruses and abnormal cells, as well as helper and suppressor cells that control the immune response by signaling the production of B cells and macrophages.

Virulence: The degree of disease-causing potential of a species of microorganism or virus as indicated by case fatality rates and/or the ability of the invader to penetrate the tissues of the host and cause disease.

Notes

Introduction: What Is Super Immunity?

1. National Intelligence Council. The global infectious disease threat and its implications for the United States. January 2000; NIE 99–17D. http://www.dni.gov/nic/special_globalinfectious.html.

2. Global alert and response: cumulative number of reported probable cases of severe acute respiratory syndrome (SARS). http://www.who.int/csr/sars/country/en/index.html.

3. Fisher ES, Wennberg DE, Stukel TA. The implications of regional variations in Medicare spending. Ann Int Med 2003; 138(4): 288–98.

4. Velicer CM, Heckbert SR, Lampe JW, et al. Antibiotic use in relation to the risk of breast cancer. JAMA 2004; 291(7): 827–35.

Chapter 1: Food Equals Health

1. Boggs DA, Palmer JR, Wise LA, et al. Fruit and vegetable intake in relation to risk of breast cancer in the Black Women's Health Study. Am J Epidemiol 2010; DOI:10.1093/aje/kwq293. Gullett NP, Ruhul Amin AR, Bayraktar S, et al. Cancer prevention with natural compounds. Semin Oncol 2010; 37(3): 258–81.

2. Li C, Ford ES, Zhao G, et al. Serum alpha-carotene concentrations and risk of death among U.S. adults. Third national Health and Nutrition Examination Survey follow-up study. Arch Intern Med 2010, Nov 22; DOI:10.1001/archinternmed.2010.440.

3. Robbins J. *Healthy at 100*. Ballantine Books, 2007.

4. Liu RH. Potential synergy of phytochemicals in cancer prevention: mechanism of action. J Nutr 2004; 134(12 Suppl): 3479S–3485S.

5. Hoover's directories: fast food and quick service restaurants 2005; www.hoovers.com/industry/fast_food_quick_service_restaurants/1444_1.html.

6. Steinmetz KA, Potter JD. Vegetables, fruit, and cancer prevention: a review. J Am Diet Assoc 1996, Oct; 96(10): 1027–39.

7. http://www.who.int/whr/1996/media_centre/press_release/en/index.html.

8. Sripaipan T, Schroeder DG, Marsh DR, et al. Effect of an integrated nutrition program on child morbidity due to respiratory infection and diarrhea in northern Viet Nam. Food Nutr Bull 2002; 23(4): 70–77.

9. Taylor CE, Higgs ES. Micronutrients and infectious diseases: thoughts on integration of mechanistic approaches into micronutrient research. J Infect Dis 2000, Sep; 182(1 Suppl): S1–S4.

10. Keusch GT. The history of nutrition: malnutrition, infection, and immunity. J Nutr 2003; 133: 336S–340S.

11. Peterhans E. Oxidants and antioxidants in viral diseases: disease mechanisms and metabolic regulation. J Nutr 1997; 127: 962S–965S.

12. Beck MA. Antioxidants and viral infections: host immune response and viral pathogenicity. J Am Coll Nutr 2001; 20(5 Suppl): 384S–388S, discussion 396S–397S.

13. Peterhans E. Oxidants and antioxidants in viral diseases mechanisms and metabolic regulation. J Nutr 1997; 127: 962S–965S.

14. Dreyfuss ML, Fawzi WW. Micronutrients and vertical transmission of HIV–1. Am J Clin Nutr 2002; 75(6): 959–70.

15. Domingo E. Newly emerging viral diseases: what role for nutrition? J Nutr 1999; 127: 958S–961S.

16. Román GC. An epidemic in Cuba of optic neuropathy, sensorineural deafness, peripheral sensory neuropathy, and dorsolateral myeloneuropathy. J Neurol Sci 1994; 127: 11–28.

17. Reid AH, Taubenberger JK, Fanning TG. The 1918 Spanish influenza: integrating history and biology. Microbes Infect 2001; 3(1): 81–87. Afkhami A. Compromised constitutions: the Iranian experience with the 1918 influenza pandemic. Bull Hist Med 2003; 77(2): 367–92.

Chapter 2: The Failure of Modern Medicine

1. Achievements in public health, 1900–1999: control of infectious diseases. MMWR 1999; 48(29): 621–29.

2. McManus IC. Life expectation of Italian Renaissance artists. Lancet 1975; 1(7901): 266–67.

3. Baicker K, Chandra A. Health affairs (2004): Medicare spending, the physician workforce, and beneficiaries' quality of care; DOI:10.1377/hlthaff .w4.184. Abramson J. Overdosed America: The Broken Promise of American Medicine. HarperCollins, 2004.

4. Tzoulaki I, Molokhia M, Curcin V, et al. Risk of cardiovascular disease and all cause mortality among patients with type 2 diabetes prescribed oral anti-diabetes drugs: retrospective cohort study using UK general practice research database. BMJ 2009; 339: b4731; DOI:10.1136/bmj.b4731. Pantalone KM, Kattan MW, Yu C, et al. The risk of developing coronary artery disease or congestive heart failure, and overall mortality, in type 2 diabetic patients receiving rosiglitazone, pioglitazone, metformin, or sulfonylureas: a retrospective analysis. Acta Diabetol 2009; 46(2): 145–54.

5. Bowker SL, Majumdar SR, Veugelers P, Johnson JA. Increased cancer-related mortality for patients with type 2 diabetes who use sulfonylureas or insulin. Diab Care 2006; 29(2): 254–58.

6. Gerstein HC, Miller ME, Byington RP, et al. Effects of intensive glucose lowering in type 2 diabetes. N Eng J Med 2008; 358(24): 254559.

7. Sipahi I, Debanne SM, Rowland DY, et al. Angiotensin-receptor blockade and risk of cancer: meta-analysis of randomized controlled trials. Lancet Oncol 2010, Jul; 11(7): 627–36.

8. US Food and Drug Administration. Benicar (olmesartan): ongoing safety review. http://www.fda.gov/Safety/MedWatch/SafetyInformation/SafetyAlerts forHumanMedicalProducts/ucm215249.htm.

9. POISE Study Group. Effects of extended-release metoprolol succinate in patients undergoing non-cardiac surgery (POISE trial): a randomized controlled trial. Lancet 2008; DOI:10.1016/S0140–6736(08) 60601–7.

10. Bangalore S, Messerli FH, Kostis JB, Pepine CJ. Cardiovascular protection using beta-blockers. J Am Coll Cardiol 2007; 50(7): 563–72.

11. Wiysonge CS, Bradley H, Mayosi BM, et al. Beta-blockers for hypertension. Cochrane Database Syst Rev 2007; (1): CD002003.

12. Swaminathan RV, Alexander KP. Pulse pressure and vascular risk in the elderly: associations and clinical implications. Am J Geriatr Cardiol 2006; 15(4): 226–32; quiz 133–34.

13. Mitchell GF, Vasan RS, Keyes MJ, et al. Pulse pressure and risk of new-onset atrial fibrillation. JAMA 2007; 297(7): 709–15.

14. Messerli FH, Mancia G, Conti CR, Hewkin AC, Kupfer S, Champion A, Kolloch R, Benetos A, Pepine CJ. Dogma disputed: can aggressively lowering blood pressure in hypertensive patients with coronary artery disease be dangerous? Ann Intern Med 2006, Jun 20; 144(12): 884–93.

15. Agency for Healthcare Research and Quality. Medication-related adverse outcomes in U.S. hospitals and emergency departments: healthcare cost and utilization project statistical brief 109; 2008, Apr. www.hcup-us.ahrq.gov/reports/statbriefs/sb109.pdf.

16. Estimates of deaths associated with seasonal influenza—United States, 1976–2007. Morbidity and Mortality Weekly Report (MMWR) 2010; 59(33); 1057–62.

17. Jefferson T, Di Pietrantonj C, Rivveti A, et al. Vaccines for preventing influenza in healthy adults. Cochrane Database Syst Rev 2010; (7): CD001269.

18. Jefferson T, Rivetti A, Hamden AR, et al. Vaccines for preventing influenza in healthy children. Cochrane Database Syst Rev 2008; (2): CD004879.

19. Jefferson T, Di Pietrantonj C, Al-Ansary LA, et al. Vaccines for preventing influenza in the elderly. Cochrane Database Syst Rev 2010; (2): CD004876.

20. Cauchon D. FDA advisers tied to industry. USA Today 2000, Sep 25. Chairman Dan Burton. Opening statement. Committee on government teform. FACA: Conflicts of interest and vaccine development: preserving the integrity of the process. 2000, Jun 15. 2154 Rayburn House Office Building, Washington, DC 20515.

21. Watanabe T. Henoch-Schonlein purpura following influenza vaccinations during the pandemic of influenza A (H1N1). Pediatr Nephrol 2011; 26(5): 795–98.

Chapter 3: Super Foods for Super Immunity

1. Amadori D, Sansoni E, Amadori A. Ovarian cancer: natural history and metastatic pattern. Front in Biosc 1996; (1): 56–59.

2. Stidley CA, Picchi MA, Leng S, et al. Multivitamins, folate, and green vegetables protect against gene promoter methylation in the aerodigestive tract of smokers. Cancer Res 2010, Jan 15; 70(2): 568–74.

3. See, for example, Yuasa Y, Nagasaki H, Akiyama Y, et al. Relationship between CDX2 gene methylation and dietary factors in gastric cancer patients. Carcinog 2005; 26(1): 193–200.

4. Walters DG, Young PJ, Agus C, et al. Cruciferous vegetable consumption alters the metabolism of the dietary carcinogen 2-amino-1-methyl-6-phenylimidazo [4,5-b]pyridine (PhIP) in humans. Carcinog 2004; 25: 1659–69.

5. Higdon JV Delage B, Williams DE, et al. Cruciferous vegetables and human cancer risk: epidemiologic evidence and mechanistic basis. Pharma Res 2007, Mar; 55(3): 224–36.

6. Brandi G, Schiavano GF, Zaffaroni N, et al. Mechanisms of action and antiproliferative properties of Brassica oleracea juice in human breast cancer cell lines. J Nutr 2005; 135(6): 1503–09. Gamet-Payrastre I, Li P, Lumeau S, et al. Sulforaphane, a naturally occurring isothiocyanate, induces cell cycle arrest and apoptosis in HT29 human colon cancer cells. Cancer Res 2000; 60: 1426–33.

7. Yuan F, Chen DZ, Liu K, et al. Anti-estrogenic activities of indole-3-carbinol in cervical cells: implication for prevention of cervical cancer. Anticancer Res 1999, May–Jun; 19(3a): 1673–80. Dalessandri KM, Firestone GL, Fitch MD, et al. Pilot study: effect of 3,3'-diindolylmethane supplements on urinary hormone metabolites in postmenopausal women with a history of early-stage breast cancer. Nutr Cancer 2004; 50: 161–67.

8. Michaud DS, Spiegelman D, Clinton SK, et al. Fruit and vegetable intake and incidence of bladder cancer in a male prospective cohort. J Natl Cancer Inst 1999; 91(7): 605–13.

9. Cohen JH, Kristal AR, Stanford JL. Fruit and vegetable intake and prostate cancer risk. J Natl Cancer Inst 2000; 92(1): 61–68.

10. Larsson SC, Hakansson N, Naslund I, et al. Fruit and vegetable consumption in relation to pancreatic cancer: a prospective study. Cancer Epidemiol Biomark Prev 2006; 15: 301–5.

11. Xue L, Pestka JJ, Li M, et al. 3,3'-diindolylmethane stimulates murine immune function in vitro and in vivo. J Nutr Biochem 2008; 19(5): 336–44.

12. Zeligs MA, Sepkovic DW, Manrique C. et al. Absorption-enhanced 3,3'-diindolylmethane: human use in HPV-related, benign, and pre-cancerous conditions. Proc Am Assoc Cancer Res 2003; 44: 3198.

13. Conrad A, Bauer D, Nobis T, et al. In vitro activity of a mixture of mustard oils (isothiocyanates) against antimicrobial and multidrug-resistant bacteria. 18th European Congress of Clinical Microbiology and Infectious Diseases 2008, Apr 19; Barcelona, Spain. Abstract number: P614.

14. Fahey JW, Haristoy X, Dolan PM, et al. Sulforaphane inhibits extracellular, intracellular, and antibiotic-resistant strains of Helicobacter pylori and prevents benzo[a]pyrene-induced stomach tumors. Proc Natl Acad Sci 2002; 99(11): 7610–15. Haristoy X, Angioi-Duprez K, Duprez A, Lozniewski A. Efficacy of sulforaphane in eradicating Helicobacter pylori in human gastric xenografts implanted in nude mice. Antimicrob Agents Chemother 2003; 47(12): 3982–84. Galan MV, Kishan AA, Silverman AL. Oral broccoli sprouts for the treatment of Helicobacter pylori infection: a preliminary report. Dig Dis Sci 2004; 49(7–8): 1088–90.

15. Zakkar M, Van der Heiden KI, Luong LA, et al. Activation of Nrf2 in endothelial cells protects arteries from exhibiting a proinflammatory state. Arteriosc Thromb & Vasc Biol 2009; 29: 1851.

16. Kohno K, Miyake M, Sano O, et al. Anti-inflammatory and immunomodulatory properties of 2-amino-3H-phenoxazin-3-one. Biol Pharma Bull 2008; 31: 1938–45. Lee JS, Park SY, Thapa D, et al. Grifola frondosa water extract alleviates intestinal inflammation by suppressing TNF-alpha production and its signaling. Exp Mol Med 2010; 42: 143–54.

17. Borchers AT, Keen CL, Gershwin ME. Mushrooms, tumors, and immunity: an update. Exp Biol Med 2004; 229: 393–406. Borchers AT, Krishnamurthy A, Keen CL, et al. The immunobiology of mushrooms. Exp Biol Med 2008; 233: 259–76.

18. Martin KR, Brophy SK. Commonly consumed and specialty dietary mushrooms reduce cellular proliferation in MCF–7 human breast cancer cells. Exp Biol Med 2010; 235: 1306–14. Fang N, Li Q, Yu S, et al. Inhibition of growth and induction of apoptosis in human cancer cell lines by an ethyl acetate fraction from shiitake mushrooms. J Altern Complement Med 2006; 12: 125–32. Ng ML, Yap AT. Inhibition of human colon carcinoma development by lentinan from shiitake mushrooms (Lentinus edodes). J Altern Complement Med 2002; 8: 581–89. Adams LS, Phung S, Wu X, et al. White button mushroom (Agaricus bisporus) exhibits antiproliferative and proapoptotic properties and inhibits prostate tumor growth in athymic mice. Nutr Cancer 2008; 60: 744–56. Lakshmi B, Ajith TA, Sheena N, et al. Antiperoxidative, anti-inflammatory, and antimutagenic activities of ethanol extract of the mycelium of Ganoderma lucidum occurring in South India. Teratog Carcinog Mutagen 2003; (1 Suppl): 85–97. Cao QZ, Lin ZB. Antitumor and anti-angiogenic activity of Ganoderma lucidum polysaccharides peptide. Acta Pharma Sinica 2004; 25: 833–38. Lin ZB, Zhang HN. Anti-tumor and immunoregulatory activities of

Ganoderma lucidum and its possible mechanisms. Acta Pharma Sinica 2004; 25: 1387–95.

19. Yu L, Fernig DG, Smith JA, et al. Reversible inhibition of proliferation of epithelial cell lines by Agaricus bisporus (edible mushroom) lectin. Cancer Res 1993; 53: 4627–32. Carrizo ME, Capaldi S, Perduca M, et al. The antineoplastic lectin of the common edible mushroom (Agaricus bisporus) has two binding sites, each specific for a different configuration at a single epimeric hydroxyl. Journal Biol Chem 2005; 280: 10614–623.

20. Hong SA, Kim K, Nam SJ, et al. A case-control study on the dietary intake of mushrooms and breast cancer risk among Korean women. Int J Cancer 2008; 122: 919–23. Shin A, Kim J, Lim SY, et al. Dietary mushroom intake and the risk of breast cancer based on hormone receptor status. Nutr Cancer 2010; 62: 476–83. Zhang M, Huang J, Xie X, et al. Dietary intakes of mushrooms and green tea combine to reduce the risk of breast cancer in Chinese women. Int J Cancer 2009; 124: 1404–08.

21. Hara M, Hanaoka T, Kobayashi M, et al. Cruciferous vegetables, mushrooms, and gastrointestinal cancer risks in a multicenter, hospital-based case-control study in Japan. Nutr Cancer 2003; 46: 138–47.

22. Chen S, Oh S, Phung S et al. Anti-aromatase activity of phytochemicals in white button mushrooms (Agaricus bisporus). Cancer Res 2006; 66(24): 12026–034.

23. Chen S, Oh SR, Phung S, et al. Anti-aromatase activity of phytochemicals in white button mushrooms (Agaricus bisporus). Cancer Res 2006; 66: 12026–034. Su B, Wong C, Hong Y, et al. Growth factor signaling enhances aromatase activity of breast cancer cells via post-transcriptional mechanisms. J Steroid Biochem Molec Biol 2011; 123: 101–8.

24. Burstein HJ, Prestrud AA, Seidenfeld J, et al. American Society of Clinical Oncology clinical practice guideline: update on adjuvant endocrine therapy for women with hormone receptor-positive breast cancer. J Clin Oncol 2010; 28: 3784–96. Riemsma R, Forbes CA, Kessels A, et al. Systematic review of aromatase inhibitors in the first-line treatment for hormone sensitive advanced or metastatic breast cancer. Breast Cancer Res Treat 2010; 123: 9–24.

25. Grube BJ, Eng ET, Kao YC, et al. White button mushroom phytochemicals inhibit aromatase activity and breast cancer cell proliferation. J Nutr 2001; 131: 3288–93.

26. Ren Z, Guo Z, Meydani SN, et al. White button mushroom enhances maturation of bone marrow-derived dendritic cells and their antigen presenting function in mice. J Nutr 2008; 138(3): 544–50.

27. Kim HJ, Barajas B, Wang M, et al. Nrf2 activation by sulforaphane restores the age-related decrease of T(H)1 immunity: role of dendritic cells. J Allergy Clin Immunol 2008; 121(5): 1255–61.

28. Yoon M, Lee J, Choi B, et al. Apigenin inhibits immunostimulatory function of dendritic cells: implication of immunotherapeutic adjuvant. Molec Pharma 2006; 70(3): 1033–44.

29. National Cancer Institute. Angiogenesis inhibitors therapy. http://www.cancer.gov/cancertopics/factsheet/Therapy/angiogenesis-inhibitors.

30. Pool-Zobel BL, Schmezer P, Sinrachatanant Y, et al. Mutagenic and genotoxic activities of extracts derived from the cooked and raw edible mushroom Agaricus bisporus. J Cancer Res Clin Oncol 1990; 116: 475–79. Toth B, Erickson J. Cancer induction in mice by feeding of the uncooked cultivated mushroom of commerce Agaricus bisporus. Cancer Res 1986; 46: 4007–11. Toth B, Erickson J, Gannett P. Lack of carcinogenesis by the baked mushroom Agaricus bisporus in mice: different feeding regimen [corrected]. In Vivo 1997; 11: 227–31.

31. Rupnick MA, Panigrahy D, Zhang CY, et al. Adipose tissue mass can be regulated through the vasculature. Proc Natl Acad Sci 2002; 99: 10730–735. Cao Y. Adipose tissue angiogenesis as a therapeutic target for obesity and metabolic diseases. Nature Rev Drug Disc 2010; 9: 107–15. Lijnen HR. Angiogenesis and obesity. Cardiovasc Res 2008; 78: 286–93. Aoki N, Yokoyama R, Asai N, et al. Adipocyte-derived microvesicles are associated with multiple angiogenic factors and induce angiogenesis in vivo and in vitro. Endocrinol 2010; 151: 2567–76.

32. Seyfi P, Mostafaie A, Mansouri K, et al. In vitro and in vivo anti-angiogenesis effect of shallot (Allium ascalonicum): a heat-stable and flavonoid-rich fraction of shallot extract potently inhibits angiogenesis. Toxicol in Vitro 2010; 24: 1655–61. Jung SK, Lee KW, Byun S, et al. Myricetin inhibits UVB-induced angiogenesis by regulating PI-3 kinase in vivo. Carcinog 2010; 31: 911–17. Powolny A, Singh S. Multitargeted prevention and therapy of cancer by diallyl trisulfide and related Allium vegetable–derived organosulfur compounds. Cancer Lett 2008; 269: 305–14.

33. Nandakumar V, Singh T, Katiyar SK. Multi-targeted prevention and therapy of cancer by proanthocyanidins. Cancer Lett 2008; 269: 378–87. Wang LS, Hecht SS, Carmella SG, et al. Anthocyanins in black raspberries prevent esophageal tumors in rats. Cancer Prev Res 2009; 2: 84–93. Stoner GD, Wang LS, Casto BC. Laboratory and clinical studies of cancer chemoprevention by antioxidants in berries. Carcinog 2008; 29: 1665–74. Roy S, Khanna S, Alessio HM, et al. Anti-angiogenic property of edible berries. Free Radic Res 2002; 36: 1023–31.

34. Hui C, Bin Y, Xiaoping Y, et al. Anticancer activities of an anthocyanin-rich extract from black rice against breast cancer cells in vitro and in vivo. Nutr Cancer 2010; 62: 1128–36.

35. Lu J, Zhang K, Nam S, et al. Novel angiogenesis inhibitory activity in cinnamon extract blocks VEGFR2 kinase and downstream signaling. Carcinog 2010; 31: 481–88.

36. Kunimasa K, Ikekita M, Sato M, et al. Nobiletin, a citrus polymethoxy-flavonoid, suppresses multiple angiogenesis-related endothelial cell functions and angiogenesis in vivo. Cancer Sci 2010; 101: 2462–69. Ashino H, Shimamura M, Nakajima H, et al. Novel function of ascorbic acid as an angiostatic factor. Angiogen 2003; 6: 259–69.

37. Cavell BE, Syed Alwi SS, Donlevy A, et al. Anti-angiogenic effects of dietary isothiocyanates: mechanisms of action and implications for human health. Biochem Pharma 2011; 81: 327–36. Kunimasa K, Kobayashi T, Kaji K, et al. Antiangiogenic effects of indole-3-carbinol and 3,3'-diindolylmethane are associated with their differential regulation of ERK1/2 and Akt in tube-forming HUVEC. J Nutr 2010; 140: 1–6. Davis R, Singh KP, Kurzrock R, et al. Sulforaphane inhibits angiogenesis through activation of FOXO transcription factors. Oncol Rep 2009; 22: 1473–78. Kumar A, D'Souza SS, Tickoo S, et al. Antiangiogenic and proapoptotic activities of allyl isothiocyanate inhibit ascites tumor growth in vivo. Integr Cancer Ther 2009; 8: 75–87.

38. Bergman Jungestrom M, Thompson LU, Dabrosin C. Flaxseed and its lignans inhibit estradiol-induced growth, angiogenesis, and secretion of vascular endothelial growth factor in human breast cancer xenografts in vivo. Clin Cancer Res 2007; 13: 1061–67.

39. Kim EC, Min JK, Kim TY, et al. [6]-Gingerol, a pungent ingredient of ginger, inhibits angiogenesis in vitro and in vivo. Biochem Biophys Res Commun 2005; 335: 300–308.

40. Liu M, Liu RH, Song BB, et al. Antiangiogenetic effects of 4 varieties of grapes in vitro. J Food Sci 2010; 75: T99–104.

41. Jung YD, Ellis LM. Inhibition of tumour invasion and angiogenesis by epigallocatechin gallate (EGCG), a major component of green tea. Int J Exp Pathol 2001; 82: 309–16. Rodriguez SK, Guo W, Liu L, et al. Green tea catechin, epigallocatechin-3-gallate, inhibits vascular endothelial growth factor angiogenic signaling by disrupting the formation of a receptor complex. Int J of Cancer 2006; 118: 1635–44. Domingo DS, Camouse MM, Hsia AH, et al. Anti-angiogenic effects of epigallocatechin-3-gallate in human skin. Int J Clin and Exp Pathol 2010; 3: 705–9. Murugan RS, Vinothini G, Hara Y, et al. Black tea polyphenols target matrix metalloproteinases, RECK, proangiogenic molecules, and histone deacetylase in a rat hepatocarcinogenesis model. Anticancer Res 2009; 29: 2301–05.

42. Lee JS, Park BC, Ko YJ, et al. Grifola frondosa (maitake mushroom) water extract inhibits vascular endothelial growth factor–induced angiogenesis through inhibition of reactive oxygen species and extracellular signal–regulated kinase phosphorylation. J Med Food 2008; 11: 643–51. Chang HH, Hsieh KY, Yeh CH, et al. Oral administration of an Enoki mushroom protein FVE activates innate and adaptive immunity and induces anti-tumor activity against murine hepatocellular carcinoma. Int Immunopharma 2010; 10: 239–46. Cao QZ, Lin ZB. Antitumor and anti-angiogenic activity of Ganoderma lucidum polysaccharides peptide. Acta Pharma Sinica 2004; 25: 833–38.

43. Szymczak M, Murray M, Petrovic N. Modulation of angiogenesis by omega-3 polyunsaturated fatty acids is mediated by cyclooxygenases. Blood 2008; 111: 3514–21.

44. Min JK, Han KY, Kim EC, et al. Capsaicin inhibits in vitro and in vivo angiogenesis. Cancer Res 2004; 64: 644–51.

45. Khan N, Afaq F, Kweon MH, et al. Oral consumption of pomegranate fruit extract inhibits growth and progression of primary lung tumors in mice. Cancer Res 2007; 67: 3475–82. Toi M, Bando H, Ramachandran C, et al. Preliminary studies on the anti-angiogenic potential of pomegranate fractions in vitro and in vivo. Angiogenesis 2003; 6: 121–28. Sartippour MR, Seeram NP, Rao JY, et al. Ellagitannin-rich pomegranate extract inhibits angiogenesis in prostate cancer in vitro and in vivo. Int J Oncol 2008; 32: 475–80.

46. Nandakumar V, Singh T, Katiyar SK. Multi-targeted prevention and therapy of cancer by proanthocyanidins. Cancer Lett 2008; 269: 378–87.

47. Kang X, Jin S, Zhang Q. Antitumor and antiangiogenic activity of soy phytoestrogen on 7,12-dimethylbenz[alpha]anthracene-induced mammary tumors following ovariectomy in Sprague-Dawley rats. J Food Sci 2009; 74: H237–42. Fotsis T, Pepper M, Adlercreutz H, et al. Genistein, a dietary-derived inhibitor of in vitro angiogenesis. Proc Natl Acad Sci 1993, 90: 2690–94.

48. Maeda N, Kokai Y, Ohtani S, et al. Anti-tumor effect of orally administered spinach glycolipid fraction on implanted cancer cells, colon–26, in mice. Lipids 2008; 43: 741–48.

49. Pannellini T, Iezzi M, Liberatore M, et al. A dietary tomato supplement prevents prostate cancer in TRAMP mice. Cancer Prev Res 2010; 3: 1284–91.

50. Bhandarkar SS, Arbiser JL. Curcumin as an inhibitor of angiogenesis. Adv Exp Med Biol 2007; 595: 185–95.

51. Szymczak M, Murray M, Petrovic N. Modulation of angiogenesis by omega-3 polyunsaturated fatty acids is mediated by cyclooxygenases. Blood 2008; 111: 3514–21. Llaverias G, Danilo C, Mercier I, et al. Role of cholesterol in the development and progression of breast cancer. Am J Path 2011; 178: 402–12. Llaverias G, Danilo C, Wang Y, et al. A Western-type diet accelerates tumor progression in an autochthonous mouse model of prostate cancer. Am J Path 2010; 177: 3180–91.

52. Powolny A, Singh S. Multitargeted prevention and therapy of cancer by diallyl trisulfide and related Allium vegetable–derived organosulfur compounds. Cancer Lett 2008; 269(2): 305–14.

53. Galeone C, Pelucchi C, Levi F, et al. Onion and garlic use and human cancer. Am J Clin Nutr 2006; 84(5): 1027–32.

54. Neurath AR, Strick N, Li YY, et al. Punica granatum (pomegranate) juice provides an HIV-1 entry inhibitor and candidate topical microbicide. BMC Infect Dis 2004; 4: 41. Jurenka JS. Therapeutic applications of pomegranate (Punica granatum L.): a review. Altern Med Rev 2008; 13(2): 128–44. Lansky EP, Newman RA. Punica granatum (pomegranate) and its potential for

264

prevention and treatment of inflammation and cancer. J Ethnopharma 2007; 109(2): 177–206.

55. Kim ND, Mehta R, Yu W, et al. Chemopreventive and adjuvant therapeutic potential of pomegranate (Punica granatum) for human breast cancer. Breast Cancer Res Treat 2002; 71(3): 203–17. Kohno H, Suzuki R, Yasui Y, et al. Pomegranate seed oil rich in conjugated linolenic acid suppresses chemically induced colon carcinogenesis in rats. Cancer Sci 2004; 95(6): 481–86. Toi M, Bando H, Ramachandran C, et al. Preliminary studies on the anti-angiogenic potential of pomegranate fractions in vitro and in vivo. Angiogen 2003; 6(2): 121–28. Kawaii S, Lansky EP. Differentiation-promoting activity of pomegranate (Punica granatum) fruit extracts in HL-60 human promyelocytic leukemia cells. J Med Food 2004; 7(1): 13–18.

56. Aviram M, Dornfeld L. Pomegranate juice consumption inhibits serum angiotensin coveting enzyme activity and reduces systolic blood pressure. Atheroscl 2001; 158(1): 195–8.

57. Aviram M, Dornfeld L, Rosenblat M, et al. Pomegranate juice consumption reduces oxidative stress, atherogenic modifications to LDL, and platelet aggregation: studies in humans and in atherosclerotic apolipoprotein E-deficient mice. Am J Clin Nutr 2000; 71(5): 1062–76.

58. Mori-Okamoto J, Otawara-Hamamoto Y, Yamato H, Yoshimura H. Pomegranate extract improves a depressive state and bone properties in menopausal syndrome model ovariectomized mice. J Ethnopharma 2004; 92(1): 93–101.

59. American Society of Nephrology (2010, Nov 19). Pomegranate juice reduces damage to tissues, inflammation, and infections, study suggests. Science Daily. Retrieved Mar 12, 2011, from http://www.sciencedaily.com/releases/2010/11/101119083126.htm.

60. Aviram M, Rosenblat M, Gaitini D, et al. Pomegranate juice consumption for 3 years by patients with carotid artery stenosis reduces common carotid intima-media thickness, blood pressure, and LDL oxidation. Clin Nutr 2004; 23(3): 423–33.

61. Adams LS, Zhang Y, Seeram NP, et al. Pomegranate ellagitannin-derived compounds exhibit antiproliferative and antiaromatase activity in breast cancer cells in vitro. Cancer Prev Res 2010; 3(1): 108–13.

62. Syed DN, Afaq F, Mukhtar H. Pomegranate derived products for cancer chemoprevention. Semin Cancer Biol 2007; 17(5): 377–85.

63. Stoner GD, Dombkowski AA, Reen RK, et al. Carcinogen-altered genes in Rat esophagus positively modulated to normal levels of expression by both black raspberries and phenylethyl isothiocyanate. Cancer Res 2008; 68(15): 6460–67.

64. Ravoori S, Kausar H, Aqil F, et al. Distinct molecular targets of blueberry and black raspberry in breast cancer prevention. Cancer Res 2010; 70(8): S1.

65. Hu FB, Stampfer MJ, Manson JE, et al. Frequent nut consumption and risk of coronary heart disease in women: prospective cohort study. BMJ 1998;

317(7169): 1341–45. Albert CM, Gaziano JM, Willett WC, et al. Nut consumption and decreased risk of sudden cardiac death in the Physicians' Health Study. Arch Intern Med 2002; 162(12): 1382–87. Kris-Etherton PM, Hu FB, Ros E, et al. The role of tree nuts and peanuts in the prevention of coronary heart disease: multiple potential mechanisms. J Nutr 2008; 138(9): 1746S–1751S. Ellsworth JL, Kushi LH, Folsom AR. Frequent nut intake and risk of death from coronary heart disease and all causes in postmenopausal women: the Iowa Women's Health Study. Nutr Metab Cardiovasc Dis 2001; 11(6): 372–77. Sabaté J, Oda K, Ros E. Nut consumption and blood lipid levels: a pooled analysis of 25 intervention trials. Arch Intern Med 2010 May 10; 170(9): 821–27. Bes-Rastrollo M, Wedick NM, Martinez-Gonzalez MA, et al. Prospective study of nut consumption, long-term weight change, and obesity risk in women. Am J Clin Nutr 2009; 89(6): 1913–19.

66. Thompson LU, Chen JM, Li T, et al. Dietary flaxseed alters tumor biological markers in postmenopausal breast cancer. Clin Cancer Res 2005; 11(10): 3828–35.

67. Cooney RV, Custer LJ, Okinaka L, et al. Effects of dietary sesame seeds on plasma tocopherol levels. Nutr Cancer 2001; 39(1): 66–71.

68. Wu WH, Kang YP, Wang NH, et al. Sesame ingestion affects sex hormones, antioxidant status, and blood lipids in postmenopausal women. J Nutr 2006; 136(5): 1270–75.

Chapter 4: Colds and Flu—What We Need to Know

1. Linder JA, Singer DE. Desire for antibiotics and antibiotic prescribing for adults with upper respiratory tract infections. J Gen Intern Med 2003; 18(10): 795–801. Nash DR, Harman J, Wald ER, Kelleher KJ. Antibiotic prescribing by primary care physicians for children with upper respiratory tract infections. Arch Pediatr Adolesc Med 2002; 156(11): 1114–19.

2. Stone S, Gonzales R, Maselli J, Lowenstein SR. Antibiotic prescribing for patients with colds, upper respiratory tract infections, and bronchitis: a national study of hospital-based emergency departments. Ann Emerg Med 2000; 36(4): 320–27.

3. Sharp HJ, Denman D, Puumala S, Leopold DA. Treatment of acute and chronic rhinosinusitis in the United States, 1999–2002. Arch Otolaryng Head Neck Surg 2007, Mar; 133(3): 260–65.

4. DiFrancesco E. Stop treating colds with antibiotics. Infect Dis News 1992, Aug; 12. Orr PH, Scherer KS, Macdonald A, Moffatt MEK. Randomized placebo-controlled trials of antibiotics for acute bronchitis: a critical review of the literature. J Fam Pract 1993; 36: 507–12.

5. Shehab N, Patel PR, Srinivasan A, Budnitz DS. Emergency department visits for antibiotic-associated adverse events. Clin Infect Dis 2008, Sep 15; 47(6): 735–43.

6. Beringer PM, Wong-Beringer A, Rho JP. Economic aspects of antibacterial adverse effects. PharmacoEcon 1998, Jan; 13: 35–49.

7. Chang ET, Smedby KE, Hjalgrim H, et al. Medication use and risk of non-Hodgkin's lymphoma. Am J Epidemiol 2005; 162(10): 965–74.

8. Velicer CM, Heckbert SR, Lampe JW, et al. Antibiotic use in relation to the risk of breast cancer. JAMA 2004; 291: 827–35.

9. Crider KS, Cleves MA, Reefhuis J, et al. Antibacterial medication use during pregnancy and risk of birth defects: national birth defects prevention study. Arch Pediatr Adolesc Med 2009; 163(11): 978–85.

10. Belanger K, Murk W, Bracken MB. Antibiotic exposure by 6 months and asthma and allergy at 6 years: findings in a cohort of 1,401 U.S. children. Am J Epidemiol 2010; DOI:10.1093/aje/kwq400.

11. Paul IM, Yoder KE, Crowell KR, et al. Effect of dextromethorphan, diphenhydramine, and placebo on nocturnal cough and sleep quality for coughing. Pediatrics 2004; 114(1): e85-e90.

12. Sutter AI, Lemiengre M, Campbell H, Mackinnon HF. Antihistamines for the common cold. Cochrane Database Syst Rev 2003; (3): CD001267.

13. Simasek M, Blandino DA. Treatment of the common cold. Am Fam Phys 2007, Feb 15; 75(4): 515–20.

14. Mackowiak P. Benefits versus risk of the febrile response. In Mackowiak P, ed. *Fever: Basic Mechanisms and Management.* Lippincott-Raven, 1997; 279–86. Husseini RH, Sweet C, Collie MH, et al. Elevation of nasal viral levels by suppression of fever in ferrets infected with influenza viruses of differing virulence. J Infect Dis 1982; 145: 520–24.

15. Graham NM, Burrell CJ, Douglas RM, et al. Adverse effects of aspirin, acetaminophen, and ibuprofen on immune function, viral shedding, and clinical status in rhinovirus-infected volunteers. J Infect Dis 1990; 162: 1277–82. Stanley ED, Jackson GG, Panusarn C, et al. Increased virus shedding with aspirin treatment of rhinovirus infection. JAMA 1975; 231: 1248–51.

16. Graham NM, Burrell CJ, Douglas RM, et al. Adverse effects of aspirin, acetaminophen, and ibuprofen on immune function, viral shedding, and clinical status in rhinovirus-infected volunteers. J Infect Dis. 1990; 162(6): 1277–82.

17. Rennard BO, Ertl RF, Gossman GL, et al. Chicken soup inhibits neutrophil chemotaxis in vitro. Chest 2000; 118(4): 1150–57.

18. Singh M. Heated, humidified air for the common cold. Cochrane Database Syst Rev 2001; (4): CD001728. Arroll B. Non-antibiotic treatments for upper-respiratory tract infections (common cold). Respir Med 2005; 99(12): 1477–84. Moore M, Little P. Humidified air inhalation for treating croup. Cochrane Database Syst Rev 2006; (3): CD002870.

19. Guppy MP, Mickan SM, Del Mar CB. Advising patients to increase fluid intake for treating acute respiratory infections. Cochrane Database Syst Rev 2005; (4): CD004419.

20. Rabago D, Zgierska A, Mundt MJ, et al. Efficacy of daily hypertonic saline nasal irrigation among patients with sinusitis: a randomized controlled trial. J Fam Pract 2002; 51(12): 1049–55.

21. Kassel JC, King D, Spurling GK. Saline nasal irrigation for acute upper respiratory tract infections. Cochrane Database Syst Rev 2010; (3): CD006821.

22. Vickers AJ, Smith C. Homoeopathic Oscillococcinum for preventing and treating influenza and influenza-like syndromes. Cochrane Database Syst Rev 2006; (3): CD001957.

23. Douglas RM, Hemilä H, Chalker E, et al. Vitamin C for preventing and treating the common cold. Cochrane Database Syst Rev 2007; (3): CD000980.

24. Taylor JA, Weber W, Standish L, et al. Efficacy and safety of echinacea in treating upper respiratory tract infections in children: a randomized controlled trial. JAMA 2003; 290(21): 2824–30.

25. Turner RB, Bauer R, Woelkart K, et al. An evaluation of Echinacea angustifolia in experimental rhinovirus infections. N Engl J Med 2005; 353: 341–48. Yale SH, Liu K. Echinacea purpurea therapy for the treatment of the common cold: a randomized, double-blind, placebo-controlled clinical trial. Arch Intern Med 2004; 164: 1237–41.

26. Lissiman E, Bhasale AL, Cohen M. Garlic for the common cold. Cochrane Database Syst Rev 2009; (3): CD006206. Josling P. Preventing the common cold with a garlic supplement: a double-blind, placebo-controlled survey. Adv Ther 2001; 18(4): 189–93.

27. Chen Q, Ganapathy S, Singh KP, et al. Resveratrol induces growth arrest and apoptosis through activation of FOXO transcription factors in prostate cancer cells. PLoS One 2010; 5(12): e15288. Patel KR, Brown VA, Jones DJ, et al. Clinical pharmacology of resveratrol and its metabolites in colorectal cancer patients. Cancer Res 2010; 70(19): 7392–99.

28. Ghanim H, Sia CL, Korzeniewski K, et al. A resveratrol and polyphenol preparation suppresses oxidative and inflammatory stress response to a high-fat, high-carbohydrate meal. J Clin Endocrinol Metab 2011; 0: jc.2010–1812v1-jc.2010–1812.

29. Kraft TE, Parisotto D, Schempp C, Efferth T. Fighting cancer with red wine? Molecular mechanisms of resveratrol. Crit Rev Food Sci Nutr 2009; 49(9): 782–99.

30. Meydani SN, Barnett JB, Dallal GE, et al. Serum zinc and pneumonia in nursing home elderly. Am J Clin Nutr 2007; 86(4): 1167–73.

31. Fischer Walker C, Black RE. Zinc and the risk for infectious disease. Ann Rev Nutr 2004; 24: 255–75.

32. Singh M, Das RR. Zinc for the common cold. Cochrane Database Syst Rev 2011; (2): CD001364.

33. Cannell JJ, Vieth R, Umhau JC, et al. Epidemic influenza and vitamin D. Epidemiol Infect 2006; 134: 1129–40. Urashima M, Segawa T, Okazaki M, et

al. Randomized trial of vitamin D supplementation to prevent seasonal influenza A in schoolchildren. Am J Clin Nutr 2010; 91: 1255–60.

34. Yamshchikov AV, Desai NS, Blumberg HM, et al. Vitamin D for treatment and prevention of infectious diseases: a systematic review of randomized controlled trials. Endocr Pract 2009; 15: 438–49.

35. Roschek B Jr, Fink RC, McMichael MD, et al. Elderberry flavonoids bind to and prevent H1N1 infection in vitro. Phytochem 2009; 70: 1255–61.

36. Zakay-Rones Z, Thom E, Wollan T, Wadstein J. Randomized study of the efficacy and safety of oral elderberry extract in the treatment of influenza A and B virus infections. J Int Med Res 2004; 32: 132–40. Vlachojannis JE, Cameron M, Chrubasik S. A systematic review of the sambuci fructus effect and efficacy profiles. Phytother Res 2010; 24(1): 1–8.

37. Roll S, Nocon M, Willich SN, et al. Reduction of common cold symptoms by encapsulated juice powder concentrate of fruits and vegetables: a randomized, double-blind, placebo-controlled trial. Brit J Nutr 2011; 105: 118–22.

38. Barringer TA, Kirk JK, Santaniello AC. Effect of a multivitamin and mineral supplement on infection and quality of life: a randomized, double-blind, placebo-controlled trial. Ann Intern Med 2003; 138(5): 365–71.

Chapter 5: Healthy Carbs, Fats, and Proteins

1. Lanza E, Hartman TJ, Albert PS, et al. High dry bean intake and reduced risk of advanced colorectal adenoma recurrence among participants in the polyp prevention trial. J Nutr 2006; 136: 1896–903. Finley JW, Burrell JB, Reeves PG, et al. Pinto bean consumption changes SCFA profiles in fecal fermentations, bacterial populations of the lower bowel, and lipid profiles in blood of humans. J Nutr 2007; 137(11): 2391–98.

2. Sluijs I, van der Schouw YT, van der A DL, et al. Carbohydrate quantity and quality and risk of type 2 diabetes in the European Prospective Investigation into Cancer and Nutrition-Netherlands (EPIC-NL) study. Am J Clin Nutr 2010; 92(4): 905–11. Barclay AW, Petocz P, McMillan-Price J, et al. Glycemic index, glycemic load, and chronic disease risk—a meta-analysis of observational studies. Am J Clin Nutr 2008, Mar; 87(3): 627–37. Gnagnarella P, Gandini S, La Vecchia C, et al. Glycemic index, glycemic load, and cancer risk: a meta-analysis. Am J Clin Nutr 2008; 87: 1793–801. Sieri S, Krogh V, Berrino F, et al. Dietary glycemic load and index and risk of coronary heart disease in a large Italian cohort: the EPICOR study. Arch Intern Med 2010; 170: 640–47. Buyken AE, Toeller M, Heitkamp G, et al. Glycemic index in the diet of European outpatients with type 1 diabetes: relations to glycated hemoglobin and serum lipids. Am J Clin Nutr 2001; 73(3): 574–81.

3. Larsson SC, Bergkvist L, Wolk A. Glycemic load, glycemic index, and breast cancer risk in a prospective cohort of Swedish women. Int J Cancer 2009, Jul 1; 125(1): 153–57. Wen W, Shu XO, Li H, et al. Dietary carbohydrates, fiber, and breast cancer risk in Chinese women. Am J Clin Nutr 2009, Jan; 89(1): 283–89. Pisani P. Hyper-insulinaemia and cancer, meta-analyses

of epidemiological studies. Arch Physiol Biochem 2008, Feb; 114(1): 63–70. Rossi M, Lipworth L, Polesel J, et al. Dietary glycemic index and glycemic load and risk of pancreatic cancer: a case-control study. Ann Epidemiol 2010, Jun; 20(6): 460–65. Thompson CL, Khiani V, Chak A, et al. Carbohydrate consumption and esophageal cancer: an ecological assessment. Am J Gastroenterol 2008, Mar; 103(3): 555–61. Augustin LS, Gallus S, Negri E, La Vecchia C. Glycemic index, glycemic load, and risk of gastric cancer. Ann Oncol 2004, Apr; 15(4): 581–84.

4. Brown MJ, Ferruzzi MG, Nguyen ML, et al. Carotenoid bioavailability is higher from salads ingested with full-fat than with fat-reduced salad dressings as measured with electrochemical detection. Am J Clin Nutr 2004; 80(2): 396–403.

5. Hu FB, Stampfer MJ. Nut consumption and risk of coronary heart disease: a review of epidemiologic evidence. Curr Atheroscler Rep 1999 Nov; 1(3): 204–9. Mukuddem-Petersen J, Oosthuizen W, Jerling JC. A systematic review of the effects of nuts on blood lipid profiles in humans. J Nutr 2005; 135(9): 2082–89. Lamarche B, Desroche S, Jenkins DJ, et al. Combined effects of a dietary portfolio of plant sterols, vegetable protein, viscous fiber, and almonds on LDL particle size. Br J Nutr 2004; 92(4): 654–63.

6. Cerda B, Tomas-Barberan FA, Espin JC. Metabolism of antioxidant and chemopreventive ellagitannins from strawberries, raspberries, walnuts, and oak-aged wine in humans: identification of biomarkers and individual variability. J Agric Food Chem 2005; 53(2): 227–35. Ros E, Naatez I, Parez-Heras A, et al. A walnut diet improves endothelial function in hypercholesterolemic subjects: a randomized crossover trial. Circulation 2004; 109(13): 1609–14.

7. Hu FB, Willett WC. Optimal diets for prevention of coronary heart disease. JAMA 2002; 288(20): 2569–78. Sabaté J. Nut consumption, vegetarian diets, ischemic heart disease risk, and all-cause mortality: evidence from epidemiologic studies. Am J Clin Nutr 1999, Sep; 70 (3): 500S–503S.

8. Ellsworth JL, Kushi LH, Folsom AR. Frequent nut intake and risk of death from coronary heart disease and all causes in postmenopausal women: the Iowa Women's Health Study. Nutr Metab Cardiovasc Dis 2001; 11(6): 372–77.

9. Coates AM, Howe PR. Edible nuts and metabolic health. Curr Opin Lipidol 2007; 18(1): 25–30. Segura R, Javierre C, Lizarraga MA, Ros E. Other relevant components of nuts: phytosterols, folate, and minerals. Br J Nutr 2006; 96(2 Suppl): S36–44.

10. Rajaram S, Sabate J. Nuts, body weight, and insulin resistance. Br J Nutr 2006; 96(2 Suppl): S79–86. Sabat ÃJ. Nut consumption and body weight. Am J Clin Nutr 2003; 78(3 Suppl): 647S–650S. Bes-Rastrollo M, Sabat ÃJ, Gamez-Gracia E, et al. Nut consumption and weight gain in a Mediterranean cohort: the SUN study. Obesity 2007; 15(1): 107–16. Garca-Lorda P, Megias Rangil I, Salas-Salvada J. Nut consumption, body weight, and insulin resistance. Eur J Clin Nutr 2003; 57(1 Suppl): S8–11. Megas-Rangil I, Garca-Lorda P, Torres-Moreno

M, et al. Nutrient content and health effects of nuts. Arch Latinoam Nutr 2004; 54(2 Suppl): 83–86.

11. Baron S, Rinsky R. NIOSH mortality study of NFL football players: 1959–88. Centers for Disease Control, National Institute for Occupational Safety and Health 1994 (HETA 88–085).

12. Gualberto A, Pollak M. Emerging role of insulin-like growth factor receptor inhibitors in oncology: early clinical trial results and future directions. Oncogene 2009; 28: 3009–21.

13. Bartke A. Minireview: role of the growth hormone/insulin-like growth factor system in mammalian aging. Endocrinol 2005; 146: 3718–23.

14. Kaaks R. Nutrition, insulin, IGF-1 metabolism, and cancer risk: a summary of epidemiological evidence. Novartis Found Symp 2004; 262: 247–60; discussion 260–68. McCarty MF. Vegan proteins may reduce risk of cancer, obesity, and cardiovascular disease by promoting increased glucagon activity. Med Hypoth 1999; 53: 459–85.

15. Cannata D, Fierz Y, Vijayakumar A, et al. Type 2 diabetes and cancer: what is the connection? Mt Sinai J Med 2010; 77: 197–213. Venkateswaran V, Haddad AQ, Fleshner NE, et al. Association of diet-induced hyperinsulinemia with accelerated growth of prostate cancer (LNCaP) xenografts. J Natl Cancer Inst 2007; 99: 1793–800.

16. Laron Z. The GH-IGF1 axis and longevity: the paradigm of IGF1 deficiency. Hormones (Athens) 2008; 7: 24–27.

17. Bonafe M, Barbieri M, Marchegiani F, et al. Polymorphic variants of insulin-like growth factor I (IGF-I) receptor and phosphoinositide 3-kinase genes affect IGF-I plasma levels and human longevity: cues for an evolutionarily conserved mechanism of life span control. J Clin Endocrinol Metab 2003; 88: 3299–304. Cheng CL, Gao TQ, Wang Z, et al. Role of insulin/insulin-like growth factor 1 signaling pathway in longevity. World J Gastroenterol 2005; 11: 1891–95.

18. Vardy ER, Rice PJ, Bowie PC, et al. Increased circulating insulin-like growth factor–1 in late-onset Alzheimer's disease. J Alz Dis 2007; 12: 285–90. Cohen E. Countering neurodegeneration by reducing the activity of the insulin/IGF signaling pathway: current knowledge and future prospects. Exp Gerontol 2010; 5: 58–71.

19. Berryman DE, Christiansen JS, Johannsson G, et al. Role of the GH/IGF-1 axis in lifespan and healthspan: lessons from animal models. Growth Horm IGF Res 2008; 18: 455–71.

20. Werner H, Bruchim I. The insulin-like growth factor-I receptor as an oncogene. Arch Physiol Biochem 2009; 115: 58–71. Chitnis MM, Yuen JS, Protheroe AS, et al. The type 1 insulin-like growth factor receptor pathway. Clin Cancer Res 2008; 14: 6364–70.

21. Rinaldi S, Peeters PH, Berrino F, et al. IGF-I, IGFBP-3 and breast cancer risk in women: the European Prospective Investigation into Cancer and Nutrition (EPIC). Endocr Relat Cancer 2006; 13: 593–605.

22. Hankinson SE, Willett WC, Colditz GA, et al. Circulating concentrations of insulin-like growth factor-I and risk of breast cancer. Lancet 1998; 351: 1393–96.

23. Lann D, LeRoith D. The role of endocrine insulin-like growth factor-I and insulin in breast cancer. J Mammary Gland Biol Neoplasia 2008; 13: 371–79. Allen NE, Roddam AW, Allen DS, et al. A prospective study of serum insulin-like growth factor-I (IGF-I), IGF-II, IGF-binding protein-3 and breast cancer risk. Br J Cancer 2005; 92: 1283–87. Fletcher O, Gibson L, Johnson N, et al. Polymorphisms and circulating levels in the insulin-like growth factor system and risk of breast cancer: a systematic review. Cancer Epidemiol Biomark Prev 2005; 14: 2–19. Renehan AG, Zwahlen M, Minder C, et al. Insulin-like growth factor (IGF)-I, IGF binding protein-3, and cancer risk: systematic review and meta-regression analysis. Lancet 2004; 363: 1346–53. Shi R, Yu H, McLarty J, et al. IGF-I and breast cancer: a meta-analysis. Int J Cancer 2004; 111: 418–23. Sugumar A, Liu YC, Xia Q, et al. Insulin-like growth factor (IGF)-I and IGF-binding protein-3 and the risk of premenopausal breast cancer: a meta-analysis of literature. Int J Cancer 2004; 111: 293–97. Baglietto L, English DR, Hopper JL, et al. Circulating insulin-like growth factor-I and binding protein-3 and the risk of breast cancer. Cancer Epidemiol Biomark Prev 2007; 16: 763–68.

24. Davies M, Gupta S, Goldspink G, et al. The insulin-like growth factor system and colorectal cancer: clinical and experimental evidence. Int J Colorectal Dis 2006; 21: 201–8. Sandhu MS, Dunger DB, Giovannucci EL. Insulin, insulin-like growth factor-I (IGF-I), IGF binding proteins, their biologic interactions, and colorectal cancer. J Natl Cancer Inst 2002; 94: 972–80. Werner H, Bruchim I. The insulin-like growth factor-I receptor as an oncogene. Arch Physiol Biochem 2009; 115: 58–71.

25. Rowlands MA, Gunnell D, Harris R, et al. Circulating insulin-like growth factor peptides and prostate cancer risk: a systematic review and meta-analysis. Int J Cancer 2009; 124: 2416–29. Weiss JM, Huang WY, Rinaldi S, et al. Endogenous sex hormones and the risk of prostate cancer: a prospective study. Int J Cancer 2008; 122: 2345–50.

26. Salvioli S, Capri M, Bucci L, et al. Why do centenarians escape or postpone cancer? The role of IGF-1, inflammation, and p53. Cancer Immunol Immunother 2009; 58: 1909–17.

27. Giovannucci E, Pollak M, Liu Y, et al. Nutritional predictors of insulin-like growth factor I and their relationships to cancer in men. Cancer Epidemiol Biomark Prev 2003; 12: 84–89.

28. Thissen JP, Ketelslegers JM, Underwood LE. Nutritional regulation of the insulin-like growth factors. Endocr Rev 1994; 15: 80–101. Clemmons DR, Seek MM, Underwood LE. Supplemental essential amino acids augment the somatomedin-C/insulin-like growth factor I response to refeeding after fasting. Metabolism 1985; 34: 391–95.

29. Holmes MD, Pollak MN, Willett WC, et al. Dietary correlates of plasma insulin-like growth factor I and insulin-like growth factor binding protein 3 concentrations. Cancer Epidemiol Biomark Prev 2002; 11: 852–61.

30. Fontana L, Weiss EP, Villareal DT, et al. Long-term effects of calorie or protein restriction on serum IGF-1 and IGFBP-3 concentration in humans. Aging Cell 2008; 7: 681–87. Allen NE, Appleby PN, Davey GK, et al. The associations of diet with serum insulin-like growth factor I and its main binding proteins in 292 women meat-eaters, vegetarians, and vegans. Cancer Epidemiol Biomark Prev 2002; 11: 1441–48. Allen NE, Appleby PN, Davey GK, et al. Hormones and diet: low insulin-like growth factor-I but normal bioavailable androgens in vegan men. Br J Cancer 2000; 83: 95–97.

31. Young VR, Pellett PL. Plant proteins in relation to human protein and amino acid nutrition. Am J Clin Nutr 1994; 59: 1203S–1212S.

32. Dewell A, Weidner G, Sumner MD, et al. Relationship of dietary protein and soy isoflavones to serum IGF-1 and IGF binding proteins in the Prostate Cancer Lifestyle Trial. Nutr Cancer 2007; 58: 35–42.

33. Dewell A, Weidner G, Sumner MD, et al. Relationship of dietary protein and soy isoflavones to serum IGF-1 and IGF binding proteins in the Prostate Cancer Lifestyle Trial. Nutr Cancer 2007; 58: 35–42. Gann PH, Kazer R, Chatterton R, et al. Sequential, randomized trial of a low-fat, high-fiber diet and soy supplementation: effects on circulating IGF-I and its binding proteins in premenopausal women. Int J Cancer 2005; 116: 297–303. Khalil DA, Lucas EA, Juma S, et al. Soy protein supplementation increases serum insulin-like growth factor-I in young and old men but does not affect markers of bone metabolism. J Nutr 2002; 132: 2605–08.

34. Fuhrman J, Sarter B, Glaser D, Acocella S. Changing perceptions of hunger on a high nutrient density diet. Nutr J 2010; 9: 51; DOI:10.1186/1475-2891-9-51.

Chapter 6: Making the Right Choices

1. Key TJ, Fraser GE, Thorogood M, et al. Mortality in vegetarians and nonvegetarians: detailed findings from a collaborative analysis of 5 prospective studies. Am J Clin Nutr 1999; 70(3): 516S–524S. Key TJA, Thorogood M, Appleby PN, Burr ML. Dietary habits and mortality in 11,000 vegetarians and health conscious people: results of a 17 year follow up. BMJ 1996; 313: 775–79. Key TJ, Appleby PN, Davey GK. Mortality in British vegetarians: review and preliminary results from EPIC-Oxford. Am J Clin Nutr 2003; 78(3 Suppl): 533S–538S.

2. Robbins J. Healthy at 100. Ballantine Books, 2007.

3. Campbell TC, Junshi C. Diet and chronic degenerative diseases: perspective from China. Am J Clin Nutr 1994; 59(5 Suppl): 1153S–1161S.

4. Tucker KL, Hallfrisch J, Qiao N, et al. The combination of high fruit and vegetable and low saturated fat intakes is more protective against mortality in aging men than is either alone: the Baltimore Longitudinal Study of Aging. J Nutr 2005; 135(3): 556–61.

5. Fraser G. *Diet, Life Expectancy, and Chronic Disease.* Oxford University Press, 2003. Fraser GE, Shavlik DJ. Ten years of life: is it a matter of choice? Arch Intern Med 2001; 161: 1645–52.

6. Nieman DC, Henson DA, Austin MD, et al. Upper respiratory tract infection is reduced in physically fit and active adults. Br J Sports Med; DOI:10.1136/bjsm.2010.077875.

7. Lee I, Hsieh C, Paffenbarger RS. Exercise intensity and longevity in men. JAMA 1995; 273: 1179–84.

8. Franco OH, de Laet C, Peeters A, et al. Effects of physical activity on life expectancy with cardiovascular disease. Arch Intern Med 2005; 165(20): 2355–60.

9. Bjelakovic G, Nikolova D, Gluud LL, et al. Antioxidant supplements for prevention of mortality in healthy participants and patients with various diseases. Cochrane Database Syst Rev 2008; (2): CD007176.

10. Xu Q, Parks CG, DeRoo LA, et al. Multivitamin use and telomere length in women. Am J Clin Nutr 2009; 89(6): 1857–63.

11. Omenn GS, Goodman GE, Thornquist MD, et al. Effects of a combination of beta carotene and vitamin A on lung cancer and cardiovascular disease. N Eng J Med 1996; 334(18): 1150–55. Hennekens CH, Buring JE, Manson JE, et al. Lack of effect of long-term supplementation with beta carotene on the incidence of malignant neoplasms and cardiovascular disease. N Eng J Med 1996; 334(18): 1145–49. Albanes D, Heinonen OP, Taylor PR, et al. Alpha-tocopherol and beta-carotene supplements and lung cancer incidence in the alpha-tocopherol, beta-carotene cancer prevention study: effects of base-line characteristics and study compliance. J Nat Cancer Inst 1996; 88(21): 1560–70. Rapola JM, Virtamo J, Ripatti S, et al. Randomized trial of alpha-tocopherol and beta-carotene supplements on incidence of major coronary events in men with previous myocardial infarction. Lancet 1997; 349(9067): 1715–20.

12. Omenn GS, Goodman GE, Thornquist MD, et al. Risk factors for lung cancer and for intervention effects in CARET, the Beta-Carotene and Retinol Efficacy Trial. J Natl Cancer Inst. 1996; 88(21): 1550–9.

13. Bjelakovic G, Nikolova D, Gluud LL, et al. Mortality in randomized trials of antioxidant supplements for primary and secondary prevention. JAMA 2007; 297: 842–57.

14. Whiting SJ, Lemke B. Excess retinol intake may explain the high incidence of osteoporosis in northern Europe. Nutr Rev 1999; 57(6): 192–95.

15. Melhus H, Michaelson K, Kindmark A, et al. Excessive dietary intake of vitamin A is associated with reduced bone mineral density and increased risk of hip fracture. Ann Intern Med 1998; 129(10): 770–78.

16. Charles D, Ness AR, Campbell D, et al. Taking folate in pregnancy and risk of maternal breast cancer. BMJ 2004; 329(7479): 1375–76.

17. Stolzenberg-Solomon RZ, Chang S, Leitzmann MF, et al. Folate intake, alcohol use, and postmenopausal breast cancer risk in the Prostate, Lung, Colorectal, and Ovarian Cancer Screening Trial. Am J Clin Nutr 2006; 83(4): 895–904.

18. Whitrow MJ, Moore VM, Rumbold AR, et al. Effect of supplemental folic acid in pregnancy on childhood asthma: a prospective birth cohort study. Am J Epidemiol 2009; 170: 1486–93. Haberg SE, London SJ, Stigum H, et al. Folic acid supplements in pregnancy and early childhood respiratory health. Arch Dis Child 2009; 94: 180–84. Kallen B. Congenital malformations in infants whose mothers reported the use of folic acid in early pregnancy in Sweden: a prospective population study. Congenit Anom 2007; 47: 119–24.

19. Fife J, Raniga S, Hider PN, Frizelle FA. Folic acid supplementation and colorectal cancer risk: a meta-analysis. Colorectal Dis 2011; 13(2): 132–37.

20. Figueiredo JC, Grau MV, Haile RW, et al. Folic acid and risk of prostate cancer: results from a randomized clinical trial. J Natl Cancer Inst 2009; 101(6): 432–35.

21. Ebbing M, Bønaa KH, Nygård O, et al. Cancer incidence and mortality after treatment with folic acid and vitamin B_{12}. JAMA 2009; 302(19): 2119–26.

22. Ebbing M, Bønaa KH, Nygård O, et al. Cancer incidence and mortality after treatment with folic acid and vitamin B_{12}. JAMA 2009; 302(19): 2119–26.

23. Figueiredo JC, Grau MV, Haile RW, et al. Folic acid and risk of prostate cancer: results from a randomized clinical trial. J Natl Cancer Inst 2009, Mar 18; 101(6): 432–35. Sellers TA, Kushi LH, Cerhan JR, et al. Dietary folate intake, alcohol, and risk of breast cancer in a prospective study of postmenopausal women. Epidemiol 2001, Jul; 12(4): 420–28. Shrubsole MJ, Jin F, Dai Q, et al. Dietary folate intake and breast cancer risk: results from the Shanghai Breast Cancer Study. Cancer Res 2001, Oct 1; 61(19): 7136–41.

24. Schlotz W, Jones A, Phillips DI, et al. Lower maternal folate status in early pregnancy is associated with childhood hyperactivity and peer problems in offspring. J Child Psychol & Psych 2010, May; 51(5): 594–602.

25. Kwan ML, Jensen CD, Block G, et al. Maternal diet and risk of childhood acute lymphoblastic leukemia. Pub Health Rep 2009, Jul–Aug; 124(4): 503–14.

26. Petridou E, Ntouvelis E, Dessypris N, et al. Maternal diet and acute lymphoblastic leukemia in young children. Cancer Epidemiol Biomark Prev 2005, Aug; 14(8): 1935–39. Huncharek M, Kupelnick B. A meta-analysis of maternal cured meat consumption during pregnancy and the risk of childhood brain tumors. Neuroepidemiol 2004, Jan–Apr; 23(1–2): 78–84. Pogoda JM, Preston-Martin S, Howe G, et al. An international case-control study of maternal diet during pregnancy and childhood brain tumor risk: a histology-specific analysis by food group. Ann Epidemiol 2009, Mar; 19(3): 148–60.

27. Turnlund JR, Jacob RA, Keen CL, et al. Long-term high copper intake: effects on indexes of copper status, antioxidant status, and immune function in young men. Am J Clin Nutr 2004 Jun; 79(6): 1037–44.

28. Morris MC, Evans DA, Tangney CC, et al. Dietary copper and high saturated and trans fat intakes associated with cognitive decline. Arch Neurol 2006, Aug; 63(8): 1085–88.

29. Ascherio A, Willett WC, Rimm EB, et al. Dietary iron intake and risk of coronary disease among men. Circulation 1994; 89(3): 969–74. Morrison HI, Semenciw RM, Mao Y, et al. Serum iron and risk of fatal acute myocardial infarction. Epidemiol1994; 5(2): 243–46.

30. Clarke TB, Davis KM, Lysenko ES, et al. Recognition of peptidoglycan from the microbiota by Nod1 enhances systemic innate immunity. Nat Med 2010; 16: 228–31.

31. de Vrese M, Rautenberg P, Laue C, et al. Probiotic bacteria reduced duration and severity but not the incidence of common cold episodes in a double blind, randomized, controlled trial. Vaccine 2006; 24: 6670–74. Pregliasco F, Anselmi G, Fonte L, et al. A new chance of preventing winter diseases by the administration of symbiotic formulations. J Clin Gastroenterol 2008; 42(3 Suppl): S224-S233. Tiollier E, Chennaoui M, Gomez-Merino D, et al. Effect of a probiotics supplementation on respiratory infections and immune and hormonal parameters during intense military training. Mil Med 2007; 172: 1006–11. Kekkonen RA., Vasankari TJ, Vuorimaa T, et al. The effect of probiotics on respiratory infections and gastrointestinal symptoms during training in marathon runners. Int J Sport Nutr Exerc Metab 2007; 17: 352–63. Kekkonen RA. Lummela N, Karjalainen H, et al. Probiotic intervention has strain specific anti-inflammatory effects in healthy adults. World J Gastroenterol 2008; 14: 2029–36.

32. He FJ, MacGregor GA. A comprehensive review on salt and health and current experience of worldwide salt reduction programmes. J Hum Hypertens, 2009; 23(6): 363–84.

33. Sanders, PW. Vascular consequences of dietary salt intake. Am J Physiol Renal Physiol 2009; 297(2): 237–43. Simon, G. Experimental evidence for blood pressure-independent vascular effects of high sodium diet. Am J Hypertens 2003; 16(12): 1074–78.

34. Dickinson KM, Clifton PM, Keogh JB. Endothelial function is impaired after a high-salt meal in healthy subjects. Am J Clin Nutr 2011; 93(3): 500–505. Lin J Hu FB, Curhan GC. Association of diet with albuminuria and kidney function decline. Clin J Am Soc Nephrol 2010; 5(5): 836–43.

35. Lorenz MW, Markus HS, Bots ML, et al. Prediction of clinical cardiovascular events with carotid intima-media thickness: a systematic review and meta-analysis. Circulation 2007; 115(4): 459–67.

36. Teucher B, Dainty JR, Spinks CA, et al. Sodium and bone health: impact of moderately high and low salt intakes on calcium metabolism in postmenopausal women. J Bone Min Res 2008; 23(9): 1477–85. Heaney RP. Role of dietary sodium in osteoporosis. J Am Coll Nutr 2006; 25(3 Suppl): 271S–276S.

37. Sonnenberg, A. Dietary salt and gastric ulcer. Gut 1986; 27(10): 1138–42. Tsugane S, Sasazuki S. Diet and the risk of gastric cancer: review of epidemiological evidence. Gastr Cancer 2007; 10(2): 75–83.

38. de Wardener HE, MacGregor GA. Harmful effects of dietary salt in addition to hypertension. J Hum Hypertens 2002; 16(4): 213–23.

39. Tuomilehto J, Jousilahti P, Rastenyte D, et. al. Urinary sodium excretion and cardiovascular mortality in Finland: a prospective study. Lancet 2001; 357 (9259): 848–51.

40. Huxley R, Man Ying Lee C, Barzi F, et al. Coffee, Decaffeinated coffee, and tea consumption in relation to incident type 2 diabetes mellitus. Arch Intern Med 2009; 169(22): 2053–63.

41. Greenberg JA, Owen DR, Geliebter A. Decaffeinated coffee and glucose metabolism in young men. Diab Care 2010; 33: 278–80.

42. Pereira MA, Parker ED, Folsom AR. Coffee consumption and risk of type 2 diabetes mellitus: an 11-year prospective study of 28,812 postmenopausal women. Arch Intern Med 2006; 166: 1311–16. Van Dijk AE, Olthof MR, Meeuse JC, et al. Acute effects of decaffeinated coffee and the major coffee components chlorogenic acid and trigonelline on glucose tolerance. Diab Care 2009; 32: 1023–25.

43. Mikuls TR, Julian BA, Bartolucci A, et al. Coffee, tea, and caffeine consumption and risk of rheumatoid arthritis. Arth & Rheum 2002; 46(1): 83–91.

44. Noordzij M, Uiterwaal CS, Arends LR, et al. Blood pressure response to chronic intake of coffee and caffeine: a meta-analysis of randomized controlled trials. J Hypertens 2005; 23: 921–28. James JE. Critical review of dietary caffeine and blood pressure: a relationship that should be taken more seriously. Psychosom Med 2004; 66: 63–71.

45. Korde LA, Wu AH, Fears T, et al. Childhood soy intake and breast cancer risk in Asian American women. Cancer Epidemiol Biomark Prev 2009; 18(4): 1050–59. Lee SA, Shu XO, Li H, et al. Adolescent and adult soy food intake and breast cancer risk: results from the Shanghai Women's Health Study. Am J Clin Nutr 2009; 89(6): 1920–26. Shu XO, Jin F, Wen W, et al. Soybean intake during adolescence and subsequent risk of breast cancer among Chinese Women. Cancer Epidemiol Biomark Prev 2001; 10: 483–88.

46. Trock BJ, Hilakivi-Clarke L, Clarke R. Meta-analysis of soy intake and breast cancer risk. J Natl Cancer Inst 2006; 98(7): 459–71.

47. Wu AH, Yu MC, Tseng CC, Pike MC. Epidemiology of soy exposures and breast cancer risk. Br J Cancer 2008; 98(1): 9–14.

48. Guha N, Kwan ML, Quesenberry CP Jr, et al. Soy isoflavones and risk of cancer recurrence in a cohort of breast cancer survivors: the Life after Cancer Epidemiology study. Breast Cancer Res Treat 2009; 118(2): 395–405.

49. Hwang YW et al. Nutr Cancer 2009; 61(5): 598–606. Hwang YW, Kim SY, Jee SH, et al. Soy food consumption and risk of prostate cancer: a meta-analysis of observational studies. Nutr Cancer 2009; 61(5): 598–606.

50. Myung SK, Ju W, Choi HJ, Kim SC, Korean Meta-Analysis (KORMA) Study Group. Soy intake and risk of endocrine-related gynecological cancer: a meta-analysis. BJOG 2009; 116(13): 1697–705.

51. Davis BC, Kris-Etherton PM. Achieving optimal essential fatty acid status in vegetarians: current knowledge and practical implications. Am J Clin Nutr 2003; 78(3 Suppl): 640S–646S. Brenna, JT. Efficiency of conversion of alpha-linolenic acid to long chain n-3 fatty acids in man. Curr Opin Clin Nutr Metab Care 2002; 5(2): 127–32.

52. Giovannucci E, Pollak M, Liu Y, et al. Nutritional predictors of insulin-like growth factor I and their relationships to cancer in men. Cancer Epidemiol Biomark Prev 2003; 12: 84–89.

53. Hardell L, Andersson SO, Carlberg M, et al. Adipose tissue concentrations of persistent organic pollutants and the risk of prostate cancer. J Occup Environ Med 2006; 48: 700–707. Van Maele-Fabry G, Libotte V, Willems J, et al. Review and meta-analysis of risk estimates for prostate cancer in pesticide manufacturing workers. Cancer Caus Contr 2006; 17: 353–73. Stripp C, Overvad K, Christensen J, et al. Fish intake is positively associated with breast cancer incidence rate. J Nutr 2003; 133(11): 3664–69. Aronson KJ, Miller AB, Wollcott CG, et al. Breast adipose tissue concentrations of polychlorinated biphenyls and other organochlorines and breast cancer risk. Cancer Epidemiol Biomark Prev 2000, Jan; 9: 55. Unger M, Olsen, J. Organochlorine compounds in the adipose tissue of deceased people with and without cancer. Environ Res 1980; 23: 257–63.

54. Kaushik M, Mozaffarian D, Spiegelman D, et al. Long-chain omega-3 fatty acids, fish intake, and the risk of type 2 diabetes mellitus. Am J Clin Nutr 2009; 90: 613–20. Brasky TM, Till C, White E, et al. Serum phospholipid fatty acids and prostate cancer risk: results from the Prostate Cancer Prevention Trial. Am J Epidemiol; published ahead of print 2011, Apr 24; DOI:10.1093/aje/kwr027. Am J Epidemiol 2011; DOI:10.1093. Stripp C, Overvad K, Christensen J, et al. Fish intake is positively associated with breast cancer incidence rate. J Nutr 2003; 133(11): 3664–69.

55. Geppert J, Kraft V, Demmelmair H, Koltzko B. Docosahexaenoic acid supplementation in vegetarians effectively increases omega-3 index: a randomized trial. Lipids 2005, Aug; 40(8): 807–14.

56. Mills PK, Dodge J, Yang R. Cancer in migrant and seasonal hired farm workers. J Agromed 2009; 14(2): 185–91.

57. Bouchard MF, Bellinger DC, Wright RO, et al. Attention-deficit hyperactivity disorder and urinary metabolites of organophosphate pesticides. Pediatrics 2010; 125:e1270–e1277.

278

58. Dinis-Oliveira RJ, Remião F, Carmo H, et al. Paraquat exposure as an etiological factor of Parkinson's disease. Neurotox 2006, Dec; 27(6): 1110–22. Tanner CM, Kamel F, Ross GW, et al. Rotenone, paraquat, and Parkinson's disease. Environ Health Perspect 2011; DOI:10.1289/ehp.1002839 (online 2011, Jan 26).

59. U.S. Department of Agriculture. http://www.ams.usda.gov/AMSv1.0/nop.

60. Grinder-Pedersen L, Rasmussen SE, Bügel S, et al. Effect of diets based on foods from conventional versus organic production on intake and excretion of flavonoids and markers of antioxidative defense in humans. J Agric Food Chem 2003, Sep 10; 51(19): 5671–76. Olsson ME, Andersson CS, Oredsson S, et al. Antioxidant levels and inhibition of cancer cell proliferation in vitro by extracts from organically and conventionally cultivated strawberries. J Agric Food Chem 2006; 54(4): 1248–55.

61. Fuhrman J, Sarter B, Calabro DJ. Brief case reports of medically supervised, water-only fasting associated with remission of autoimmune disease. Altern Ther Health Med 2002, Jul–Aug; 8(4): 110–12.

62. Müller H, de Toledo FW, Resch KL, et al. Fasting followed by vegetarian diet in patients with rheumatoid arthritis: a systematic review. Scand J Rheum 2001; 30(1): 1–10. Darlington LG, Ramsey NW, Mansfield JR. Placebo-controlled, blind study of dietary manipulation therapy in rheumatoid arthritis. Lancet 1986; 1(8475): 236–38.

63. Nenonen M, Törrönen R, Häkkinen AS, et al. Antioxidants in vegan diet and rheumatic disorders. Toxicol 2000; 155(1–3): 45–53.

64. Leiba A, Armital H, Gershwin ME, Shoenfeld Y. Diet and Lupus 2001; 10(3): 246–48. McCarty MF. Upregulation of lymphocyte apoptosis as a strategy for preventing and treating autoimmune disorders: a role for whole-food vegan diets, fish oil, and dopamine agonists. Med Hypoth 2001; 57(2): 258–75.

65. Simopoulos AP. Omega-3 fatty acids in inflammation and autoimmune disease. J Am Coll Nutr 2002; 21(6): 495–505. Ergas D, Eilat E, Mendlovic S, Sthoeger ZM. n-3 fatty acids and the immune system in autoimmunity. Isr Med Assoc J 2002; 4(1): 34–38. Kelley DS. Modulation of human immune and inflammatory responses by dietary fatty acids. Nutr 2001; 17(7): 669–73.

66. Cantona MT. Vitamin D and autoimmunity: is vitamin D status an environmental factor affecting autoimmune disease prevalence? Proc Soc Exp Biol Med 2000; 223 (3): 230–33. Merlino LA, Curtis J, Mikuls TR, et al. Vitamin D intake is inversely associated with rheumatoid arthritis: results from the Iowa Women's Health Study. Arth & Rheum 2004; 50 (1): 72–77. Oelzner P, Muller A, Deschner F, et al. Relationship between disease activity and serum levels of vitamin D metabolites and PTH in rheumatoid arthritis. Calcif Tissue Int 1998 62(3): 193–98. Muller K, Kriegbaum NJ, Baslund B, et al. Vitamin D3 metabolism in patients with rheumatic diseases: low serum levels of 25-hydroxyvitamin D3 in patients with systemic lupus erythematosus. Clin Rheum 1995 14(4): 397–400.

Acknowledgments

I'd like to acknowledge my hard-working professional team. Linda Popescu, R.D., who assists me with nutritional scoring calculations and high-nutrient recipes. Deana Ferreri, Ph.D., a research scientist who works with me analyzing research. Jay Benson, D.O., who has worked overtime to lessen my workload to enable me to finish this book on schedule. Christine Waltermyer, who trialed and tweaked recipes for final taste testing. I also want to acknowledge my executive team at DrFuhrman.com—Janice Marra, Dominic Ambrosio, and Elijah Lynn—who work with tireless enthusiasm.

Index

Abramson, John, 40
acai berries, 80
acetaminophen, 95–96, 107
aging
  animal products and, 123
  cancer and, 72
  cellular telomeres and, 145–46
  dendritic cells and, 72
  free radicals and premature, 17, 66
  later life disease, reduction of, 18
  resveratrol as anti-aging, 101
  seeds/nuts for muscle-bone mass, 117
  slowing of, 8, 21
  waste products and, 110
ALA (alpha-linolenic acid), 161, 162, 164
algae, 161, 162
allergies, 6, 23, 51, 60, 88, 162
alliums, 16, 19, 75 76–77
allyl isothiocyanate (AITC), 64
allyl sulfides, 16, 19
almond(s)
  Caesar's Secret Salad, 203
  Golden Delicious Truffles, 243
  Golden Onion Morsels, 211
  Hemp Nutri-Milk, 196
  nutrient density, 27
  Peanut Ginger Dressing, 200
  piecrust, 245
  Rainbow Chopped Salad, 206
almond butter
  Aztec Stuffer, 237
  Black Bean Brownies, 239
  Mumbai Stuffer, 237
  Peanut Ginger Dressing, 200
alpha-carotene, 16, 17, 18, 34, 116
  blood test for, 17–18
  foods high in, 18, 19
alpha-lipoic acid, 16
Alzheimer's disease, 126, 162
amino acids, 81, 121, 124, 127, 128, 142
andrographis, 100
angiogenesis, 41–42, 63, 73, 73–74, 74
  dietary inhibitors, 72–73, 74, 75, 77, 78
animal products, 15, 16, 17, 20, 35, 38,
  121, 123, 137, 139
  animal vs. plant-based protein, 121–24

  avoiding, 96, 129
  Dr. Fuhrman's Food Pyramid and, 28
  foods to eliminate, 130, 177
  IGF-1 and, 124–27
  Nutrient Density Scores, 27
  toxins in, 165
  transition to fewer, 140–42
  type to choose, 133
  using safely, 130, 131–32, 136, 137, 177
  zinc in, 103
anthocyanins, 16, 19, 78, 80, 105
antibacterials, 20, 87
  dietary, 65–67, 78
antibiotics, 7, 44, 87–89
  bacterial resistance to, 65, 88, 90,
    91–92
  cancer link, 7, 87
  diseases resistant to, 30
  good bacteria and, 88, 89–92, 152, 153
  infants and, 88
  as over-prescribed, 85, 86
  pregnancy, birth defects, and, 87–88
  reasons to avoid use of, 86–88
  secondary infections and, 152–53
antihistamines, 94
anti-inflammatory foods, 63, 77, 78
  for autoimmune diseases, 172
  longevity, cancer protection, and, 127
antioxidants, 13, 16–21
  ARE and, 66–67
  dietary, 17, 77, 78, 117
  ITCs and, 63
  Nrf2 and, 66–67
  organic produce and, 167
antivirals, 20
  dietary, 65–67, 104–5
  for flu, 52
  resveratrol as, 101–2
  zinc as, 102–4
apoptosis, 21, 63
apple(s)
  Berrynut Bites, 238
  Blackberry, Surprise, 189
  Bok Choy Salad, 202
  Cinnamon, Omega Milk, 196
  Coconut Carrot Cream Pie, 242–43

apple(s) *(continued)*
  Golden Delicious Truffles, 243
  nutrient density, 27
  pesticides and, 166
  Phyto-Blast Breakfast Bowl, 191
  Powerhouse Micro Salad, 206
  Super Seed Oatmeal, 193
  Waldorf Blended Salad, 198
  Wild Blueberry Pie, 245
apricots or apricot nectar
  Berry Boost Gelatin, 238
  Golden Delicious Truffles, 243
ARE, 66–67
aromatase, 71–72, 79
arugula, 69, 82
  Mighty Mushroom Stroganoff, 230–31
  nutrient density, 27, 131
asparagus, 19
  in "Clean Fifteen," 166
  folate in, 148
  nutrient density, 27
aspirin, 94–95
asthma, 52, 60, 88
astragalus, 100
autoimmune diseases, 23, 167–73
  DHA, EPA, and, 162
  mushrooms and, 70
  nutritional intervention for, 168–72
  protocol for treatment, features of, 172
avocados
  in "Clean Fifteen," 166
  Dr. Fuhrman's Food Pyramid and, 28
  Got Greens Smoothie, 197
  health benefits of, 118
  nutrient density, 27
  Pesto Dressing, 201
  Simple Guacamole, 213

bacteria, healthy, 89–92
bananas
  Black Cherry Sorbet, 239
  Chunky Blueberry Walnut Sorbet, 241
  frozen, cream, 190
  Ginger Dressing, 199
  Go Berry Breakfast Bars, 191
  Got Greens Smoothie, 197
  nutrient density, 27
  Phyto-Blast Breakfast Bowl, 191
  Quick, Berry Breakfast to Go, 192
  Tropical Fruit Salad, 209
  Very Berry Smoothie, 198
  Wild Blueberry Hot Breakfast, 195

barley
  GI and GL of, 112
  as recommended carb, 113
  resistant starch + fiber in, 114
Barsamian, Aram, 11
basil
  Pesto Dressing, 201
  Tomato Bisque, 219
beans and legumes, 15, 23, 36
  as anticancer agent, 160
  Anticancer Soup, 216
  Black, and Corn Salsa, 210
  Black, Brownies, 239
  Black, Lettuce Bundles, 223
  Dr. Fuhrman's Food Pyramid and, 28
  Enchiladas, 221
  GI and GL of, 112
  Goji Chili Stew, 227
  immune system and, 26
  Island Black, Dip, 212
  Lisa's Lovely Lentil Stew, 229
  Mighty Mushroom Stroganoff, 230–31
  nutrient density, 27, 131
  Portobello Mushrooms and, 231
  as recommended carb, 113
  resistant starch + fiber in, 114
  servings per day, 130
  Shiitake Watercress Soup, 218
  Spaghetti Squash Primavera, 232
  Tangy White, and Zucchini, 235
  zinc in, 103
beef. *See also* animal products
  amount recommended daily, 132
  fast food burgers as dangerous, 133
  nutrient density, 27
beet(s)
  Healthy Chocolate Cake, 244
  Sweet, Potato Cakes with Strawberry
    Sauce, 194
berry(ies), 13, 82
  anthocyanins in, 105
  anticancer and immune system-enhanc-
    ing of, 59, 72, 74, 75, 79–80
  Boost Gelatin, 238
  Chocolate Dip with Fresh Fruit and,
    240–41
  ETs in, 118
  flavonoids in, 72
  Purple Power Smoothie, 198
  Quick Banana, Breakfast to Go, 192
  as recommended carb, 113
  Super Seed Oatmeal, 193

beta-carotene, 16, 17, 34, 116
  supplement caution, 146–47
betalains, 19
bioflavonoids, 16, 33, 172
Black, Debra, 170–71
blackberries, 79–80
  Apple Surprise, 189
  nutrient density, 27, 131
  Very Berry Smoothie, 198
blueberry(ies), 80
  Chocolate Dip with Fresh Fruit and
    Berries, 240–41
  Chunky, Walnut Sorbet, 241
  Forbidden Rice Pudding, 190
  Go Berry Breakfast Bars, 191
  nutrient density, 27, 131
  pesticides and, 166
  Purple Power Smoothie, 198
  Quick Banana Berry Breakfast to Go, 192
  Super Seed Oatmeal, 193
  Very Berry Smoothie, 198
  Wild, Hot Breakfast, 195
  Wild, Pie, 245
body mass index (BMI), 123–24
bok choy, 19, 69
  Apple, Salad, 202
  Detox Green Tea, 197
  nutrient density, 27, 131
  Rainbow Chopped Salad, 206
Boller, Emily, 1, 2
bone health, 123, 147, 155
breakfast
  avoiding sweetened cereals, 109, 113
  recipes, 189–95
breast cancer, 4, 25
  antibiotics linked to, 7, 87
  diabetes link, 125
  dietary anticancer agents, 26, 64, 70–72,
    78, 79, 81, 159–60
  folic acid and increased risk, 149
  insulin, IGF-1, and, 125, 126
  ITCs and, 64
  multivitamins and increased risk, 149
  sex hormones and, 125
broccoli, 19, 62, 69, 82
  anticancer effects, 63
  Easy Vegetable Pizza, 226
  folate in, 148
  Goji Chili Stew, 227
  nutrient density of, 131
  Powerhouse Micro Salad, 206
  zinc in, 103

broccolini, 69
broccoli rabe, 69
broccoli sprouts: Nutri-Green Salad with
  Black Fig Dressing, 205
bronchitis, 85, 86, 92
brussels sprouts, 69, 82
  anticancer effects, 63
  folate in, 148
  nutrient density, 27, 131
  Polonaise, 224

cabbage, 19, 62, 69, 82
  in "Clean Fifteen," 166
  Mumbai Stuffer, 237
  nutrient density, 27, 131
  Powerhouse Micro Salad, 206
  Rainbow Chopped Salad, 206
  reduction of pancreatic cancer and, 65
  Spaghetti Squash Primavera, 232
  steaming, 69
  Thai Longevity Stew, 236
  Triple Treat Cabbage Salad, 208
Caesar's Secret Salad, 203
calcium, foods high in, 81
cancer, 4, 8, 9, 14, 23–25, 38, 46
  aging and, 72
  alpha-carotene and lowered risk, 18
  angiogenesis and, 41–42, 63, 72–74
  animal products and, 137
  antibiotics link, 7, 87
  Anticancer Soup, 216
  apoptosis and, 21, 63
  ARBs and angiogenesis, 41–42
  case studies, 57–58, 60–61
  in children, 150
  DHA, EPA, and, 162
  diabetes link, 125
  DNA damage and, 61–62
  environmental factors, 56, 61
  epidemic, IGF-1 and, 125
  ETs for prevention, 118
  folate and reduced risk, 149–50
  folic acid and increased risk, 149, 150
  high-GL foods as risk factor, 112
  hormone-sensitive, 64
  immune system and, 3, 8, 56
  intake of vegetables and rates of, 19
  methylation, greens, and, 61–62
  modern diet and, 4, 20, 23
  nutritional protection from, 26, 36, 52,
    57–58, 59, 63–80, 117, 149–50, 160
  pesticides and, 164–65

cancer *(continued)*
  phytochemicals and resistance to, 20–21
  as preventable, 46
  tumor growth and IGF-1, 125, 126, 128
  vitamin A risk, 147
cantaloupe
  in "Clean Fifteen," 166
  nutrient density, 27
carbohydrates, 111–15
  fiber in healthiest, 111, 113
  GI and GL of common plant foods, 112
  glycemic index of, 111–13
  recommended foods, 113–14
  refined, and insulin production, 125
  resistant starch + fiber in common plant
    foods, 114
  rule and rhyme for, 115
  unacceptable, 114–15
cardiovascular disease. *See* heart disease
carotene/carotene family, 16, 18, 33, 116
  beta-carotene supplement caution, 146
carrots/carrot juice, 17, 19, 82
  Anticancer Soup, 216
  Apple Bok Choy Salad, 202
  Coconut, Cream Pie, 242–43
  Creamy Butternut Squash Soup with
    Mushrooms, 215
  Golden Austrian Cauliflower Cream
    Soup, 217
  Healthy Chocolate Cake, 244
  nutrient density, 27, 131
  Powerhouse Micro Salad, 206
  Rainbow Chopped Salad, 206
  Shiitake Watercress Soup, 218
  Spaghetti Squash Primavera, 232
  Thai Longevity Stew, 236
cashews
  Anticancer Soup, 216
  Apple Bok Choy Salad, 202
  Caesar's Secret Salad, 203
  Cinnamon Apple Omega Milk, 196
  Creamy Cruciferous Curry, 225
  Golden Delicious Truffles, 243
  Golden Onion Morsels, 211
  nutrient density, 27
  Orange Cashame Dressing, 200
  Peanut Ginger Dressing, 200
  Triple Treat Cabbage Salad dressing, 208
cauliflower, 62, 69
  Creamy Cruciferous Curry, 225
  Golden Austrian, Cream Soup, 217
  Mighty Mushroom Stroganoff, 230–31
  nutrient density of, 131

celery
  Anticancer Soup, 216
  Creamy Butternut Squash Soup with
    Mushrooms, 215
  pesticides and, 166
  Powerhouse Micro Salad, 206
cereals
  avoiding sweetened, 109, 113
  Pomegranate Museli, 192
  Quick Banana Berry Breakfast to Go,
    192
  Super Seed Oatmeal, 193
cervical dysplasia, 65
cheese, 15, 28. *See also* dairy products
cherry(ies)
  Black, Sorbet, 239
  Detox Green Tea, 197
  nutrient density, 27, 131
  pesticides and, 166
chia seeds, 82
  ALA in, 161
  Cookies, 240
  nutrient density, 27, 131
chicken, 15, 20, 27, 132
chickpeas
  Creamy Cruciferous Curry, 225
  Eggplant Hummus, 211
  folate in, 148
  Portobello Mushrooms and Beans, 231
children
  acetaminophen danger, 96
  cancer in, 150
  colds, frequency of, 2
  fevers and, 37, 95
  flu and, 37, 52, 54–55
  flu vaccination and, 49, 50–51
  folic acid and health problems, 150
  immunity and, 37, 52
  mercury in vaccines and, 50
  pesticides and health risks, 165
  zinc and reduction in mortality, 102
Chili Stew, Goji, 227
chlorogenic acid, 157
chocolate
  Black Bean Brownies, 239
  Dip with Fresh Fruit and Berries, 240–41
  Healthy, Cake, 244
  nut icing, 244
cholesterol
  foods to avoid, 109
  raw seeds and nuts for, 117, 118
cinnamon, 75
  Apple Omega Milk, 196

CNA (comprehensive nutritional adequacy), 31
coconut
  Carrot Cream Pie, 242–43
  Chia Cookies, 240
  Wild Blueberry Hot Breakfast, 195
coffee, 156–58
colds, 2, 5, 8, 9, 85–107
  chicken soup for, 96
  cough medications, 107
  echinacea for, 99–100
  elderberry extract for, 104–5
  exercise and fewer, 142–43
  fever and, 107
  fluid intake and, 97, 107
  food restriction and, 96, 107
  garlic for, 100
  homeopathic remedies, 98
  humidifier or steam inhaler for, 97, 107
  immune system and, 11
  mucus color and, 86, 106
  nasal saline irrigation, 97
  OTC medications for, 92–96, 107
  points to remember when ill, 106–7
  remedy review, 105–7
  resveratrol for, 101
  Super Immunity and prevention of, 89
  transmission of, 86
  viral types and, 85–86
  vitamin C and, 98–99, 107
  vitamin D for, 104
  when to call the doctor, 107
  zinc for, 102–4
collards, 19, 62, 69, 82
  Anticancer Soup, 216
  Aztec Stuffer, 237
  Green Leafy Moroccan Medley, 228
  nutrient density, 27, 131
  Sweet Beet Potato Cakes with Strawberry sauce, 194
  Waldorf Blended Salad, 198
colorectal cancers, 26
  diabetes link, 125
  dietary anticancer agents, 64, 71, 78, 79
  good bacteria as protective, 90
  IGF-1 and, 126
  ITCs and, 64
copper, 151
corn
  Bean Enchiladas, 221
  Black Bean and, Salsa, 210
  in "Clean Fifteen," 166
  GI and GL of, 112

Goji Chili Stew, 227
  nutrient density, 27
  protein content, 122
  as recommended carb, 113
  resistant starch + fiber in, 114
corn syrup, 15
coronary artery disease (CAD), 43
cough medications, 93–94
coumestans, 19
Crohn's diease, 142, 168, 249
cucumbers
  Detox Green Tea, 197
  nutrient density, 27
currants
  Blackberry Apple Surprise, 189
  Chia Cookies, 240
  Marinated Kale Salad, 204
cyanidin 3-glucoside, 105
cyanidin 3-sambubioside, 105

dairy products, 28
  amount recommended daily, 132
  foods to avoid, 130
  IGF-1 and, 127
  nutrient density, 27
  toxins in, 165
dates
  Almond Hemp Nutri-Milk, 196
  Apple Berrynut Bites, 238
  Black Bean Brownies, 239
  Chocolate Dip with Fresh Fruit and Berries, 240–41
  Healthy Chocolate Cake, 244
  Home-Style Ketchup, 212
  piecrust, 245
  Purple Power Smoothie, 198
  Strawberry Sesame Vinaigrette, 207
  Wild Blueberry Pie, 245
deficiency diseases, 22, 23
dementia, 14, 36, 83
depression, 53, 79, 162
desserts
  cookies, number daily, 132
  elimination of sweets and, 140
  homemade, 133
  recipes, 238–45
Detox Green Tea, 197
detoxification, 20, 66, 171
DHA (docosahexaenoic acid), 116, 138
  amount recommended daily, 164
  foods high in, 161, 163
  health risks of deficiency, 162
  supplements, 138, 172

diabetes
ACCORD study, 41
cancer link, 125
causes of type 2, 40–41
coffee and decreased risk, 156–57
drugs for, 40–41
foods to avoid, 109
high-GL foods as risk factor, 112
nutritional protection from, 52
DIM (diindolylmethane), 64, 65
DNA
cellular telomeres and, 145
damage and cancer, 21, 61–62
dietary protection of, 62, 70
epigenetic changes and, 62
methylation, 147
phytochemicals and, 20
repair of, 20
DrFuhrman.com, 168
Dr. Fuhrman's Famous Anticancer Soup, 216
Dr. Fuhrman's Food Pyramid, 28, 29
Dr. Fuhrman's Nutrient Density Scores, 27

echinacea, 99–100
edamame, 103, 148
eggplant
anthocyanins in, 105
in "Clean Fifteen," 166
Cremini Ratatouille, 226
Hummus, 211
Super Food Stuffed Peppers, 233
eggs, 133
amount recommended daily, 132
Dr. Fuhrman's Food Pyramid and, 28
nutrient density, 27
elderberries, 80
extract, for colds and flu, 104–5, 106
ellagic acid, 80
ellagitannins (ETs), 118
endometrial cancer, 160
EPA (eicosapentaenoic acid), 138
foods high in, 161, 163
health risks of deficiency, 162
supplements, 138, 172
esophageal cancer, 79
exercise, 142–44

fast food, 22, 23, 38, 133
fat, body. See also obesity; weight loss
angiogenesis and, 73, 73
foods that promote angiogenesis, 75

fats, dietary, 116–21. See also omega-3 fatty acids
benefits of raw seeds and nuts and, 117
best high-fat foods, 116
as dominant in modern world's diet, 35
Dr. Fuhrman's Food Pyramid and, 28
health issues and deficiency, 116–17
health problems from, 118
low-fat diet and health, 110, 117
as necessary, 25, 116–17
olive oil, misconceptions about, 119–20
percentage of diet, 110–11
saturated, 128
whole foods vs. extracted oils, 119
in wild salmon and sardines, 138
fermented foods, 152
fever, 37, 94–95, 107
when to call the doctor, 55
fiber, dietary, 111, 113, 119, 141
resistant starch + fiber in common plant foods, 114
fish
amount recommended daily, 132
clean, wild, 133
DHA/EPA in, 138–39, 161, 162, 163
farm-raised, 163
near-vegan diet and, 136
nutrient density, 27
pollutants in, 163
fish oil, 161, 163–64
flavonoids, 16, 19, 72, 105
flavonols glucosinolates, 19
flax seeds, 75, 81, 82, 119, 141, 161, 164
amount recommended daily, 164
nutrient density, 27, 131
Powerhouse Micro Salad, 206
flexitarian diet, 81, 102, 116, 177
flu, 2, 85–107. See also colds
antiviral drugs and, 52–53
in children, 37, 49
complications of, 3, 5, 47–48
elderberry extract for, 104–5
facts about, 45–46
flu shots, pro and con, 47–52
mucus color and, 86
mutation of virus, 34
1918–19 pandemic, 35–36
nutritarian diet as intervention, 34–35
nutritional status of host and, 32–33
OTC medications for, 92–96
points to remember when ill, 106–7

prevention, 54–55
remedy review, 105–7
resistance to, 8, 9
at-risk population, 51–52
Super Immunity and prevention of, 89
symptoms, 46
transmission of, 86
viral types and, 86
virulent strains, 46
vitamin D for, 104
when to call the doctor, 55
folate, 17, 33, 147–51
folic acid
    pregnancy and, 148, 149, 150
    supplement caution, 145, 147–51
    as synthetic, 148
fortification (of foods), 22–23
free radicals, 13, 16–17, 20, 66, 144
fried foods, 130
fruit juices, 109, 131
fruit(s), 15, 36
    as angiogenesis inhibitor, 75
    Chocolate Dip with Fresh, and Berries, 240–41
    citrus, 75
    color of and phytochemicals, 72
    Dirty Dozen and Clean Fifteen, 166
    Dr. Fuhrman's Food Pyramid and, 28
    immune system and, 26
    nutrient density of, 27, 131
    organic, pesticides, and, 164–67
    as recommended carb, 113
    servings per day, 130
    Tropical, Salad, 209

garlic, 82
    Caesar's Secret Salad dressing, 203
    for colds and flu, 100
    how to roast, 203
    immune system-enhancing of, 76–77
    Thai Longevity Stew, 236
gastrointestinal tract
    antibiotics and, 88, 89–92, 152, 153
    DHA, EPA, and, 162
    foods for "good" bacteria, 152
    immune system and, 89, 151–52
    inflammatory bowel disease, 162, 168
    medical conditions of, 142
    probiotics and, 152
GBOMBS, 83
ginger, 75, 172
    Banana, Dressing, 199

Peanut, Dressing, 200
Thai Longevity Stew, 236
ginseng, 100
glucosinolates, 16, 67–68, 68
glycemic index (GI), 111–13
glycemic load (GL), 112, 113
goji berries, 80
    Balsamic Dressing, 199
    Chili Stew, 227
    Chocolate Dip with Fresh Fruit and Berries, 240–41
    Marinated Kale Salad, 204
    Rainbow Chopped Salad, 206
golden seal, 100
grapefruit, 166
grapes, 75, 105, 166
    nutrient density of red, 27, 131
greens (green vegetables), 13, 25–26
    ALA in, 161
    alpha-carotene and, 18, 19
    as angiogenesis inhibitor, 74
    anticancer and immune system-enhancing of, 59, 63–65, 75
    antioxidants in, 17
    as antiviral and antibacterial, 65–67
    cruciferous, 62–69
    Green Leafy Moroccan Medley, 228
    ITCs and, 65
    methylation, cancer risk, and, 61–62
    nutrient density of, 18
    Nutri-Green Salad with Black Fig Dressing, 205
    phytochemicals in, 161
    protein in, 122
    servings per day, 130
    synergy with mushrooms, 71, 74
    weight loss and, 129
green tea, 71, 75
    Detox Green Tea, 197
growth hormone (GH), 124, 125–26
Guacamole, 213
Guillain-Barré syndrome, 48, 51

health equation, 109
heart disease, 3, 46
    angiotensin receptor blockers and, 41–42
    beta-blockers and, 42, 43
    beta-carotene caution, 146–47
    DHA, EPA, and, 162
    foods that increase risk, 109
    high-GL foods as risk factor, 112

heart disease *(continued)*
    hypertension and, 154
    increasing incidence of, 38
    iron and increased risk, 151
    low blood pressure danger, 43
    low-fat diet regimens and, 110
    Nrf2 and plaque formation, 67
    nutritional protection, 14, 18, 36, 52,
        78, 79, 83, 117, 118
Helicobacter pylori, 65–66
hemp seeds
    ALA in, 161
    Almond, Nutri-Milk, 196
    Cinnamon Apple Omega Milk, 196
    nutrient density, 27, 131
    phytochemicals in, 161
    protein in, 141
Henoch-Schonlein purpura, 51
hepatitis, 65
herpes, 34–35, 101
HIV/AIDs, 33, 34–35
    cruciferous vegetables as antivirals, 65
homeopathic remedies, 98
horseradish, 69
HPV (human papilloma virus), 65
Hummus, Eggplant, 211
hypertension (high blood pressure)
    ARBs for, 41–42
    beta-blockers for, 42
    incidence in U.S., 154
    mortality risk and, 43
    POISE trial, 42
    pomegranates for, 78
    salt and, 154
    side effects of medication, 42–43

ibuprofen, 94–95, 107
immune system, 1, 16, 36, 64, 83. *See
    also* autoimmune diseases; Super
    Immunity
    cancer and, 3, 8, 56 *(see also* cancer)
    cytotoxic power of, 20
    dendritic cells, 72
    exercise and, 142–43
    foods that strengthen, 26, 36, 59, 65–80,
        161 *(see also* Super Foods)
    frequency of colds or flu and, 1, 2
    gastrointestinal tract and, 89, 151–52
    modern diet and, 4, 20, 25
    natural killer T cells (NKT), 70
    phytochemicals and, 9, 19, 20
    viruses and, 29–32

immune system disorders, 23. *See also*
    autoimmune diseases
indoles, 19, 64, 65
infectious disease. *See also specific diseases*
    alpha-carotene and lowered risk, 18
    etiology of, 30–31
    famine and epidemic association, 36
    globalization of, 3–4
    increase of deaths from, 30
    nutritional protection from, 32–33, 36
    proliferation of new types, 3
    reducing exposure to, 31
    resistance to, 14
    U.S. death rates from, 3
    Vietnam children study, 31–32
    waste products and susceptibility, 110
influenza. *See* flu
insulin, 75, 125
insulin-like growth factor 1 (IGF-1), 124–27
interferon, 65
iodine, 22, 139, 144
iron, 22
    foods high in, 81
    supplement caution, 151
isoflavones, 19, 159
isothiocyanates, 16, 63
isothiocyanates (ITCS), 63–64, 65, 72

juniper, 100

kale, 62, 69, 82
    Anticancer Soup, 216
    Braised, and Squash with Pumpkin
        Seeds, 224
    "Cheesy," Soup, 214
    Creamy Cruciferous Curry, 225
    Marinated, Salad, 204
    nutrient density, 27, 131
    pesticides and, 166
    Seasoned, Chips and Popcorn, 213
    Waldorf Blended Salad, 198
    zinc in, 103
Kaminski, Laura, 6
kidney health, 79
kiwi
    in "Clean Fifteen," 166
    Got Greens Smoothie, 197
kohlrabi, 69

laryngeal papillomas, 65
leeks
    Anticancer soup, 216

Golden Austrian Cauliflower Cream
  Soup, 217
nutrient density, 27, 131
Shiitake Watercress Soup, 218
Thai Longevity Stew, 236
lentils
  folate in, 148
  GI and GL of, 112
  Lisa's Lovely, Stew, 229
  nutrient density, 27
  protein content, 122
lettuce, 82
  Black Bean, Bundles, 223
  Caesar's Secret Salad, 203
  Detox Green Tea, 197
  folate in Romaine, 148
  Got Greens Smoothie, 197
  Italian Stuffer, 237
  nutrient density, 27, 131
  Purple Power Smoothie, 198
  Waldorf Blended Salad, 198
leukemia, 78, 165
lignans, 16, 19, 81, 118
liminoids, 19
longevity (life expectancy)
  in adult males, 38–39
  animal products restriction and, 139
  average lifespan increase, 38
  exercise and enhanced, 143–44
  IGF-1 and, 126, 127, 129
  immune-enhancement and increased, 56
  larger BMI and early death, 123–24
  longest-living populations, 19, 38, 136
  low systemic inflammation and, 127
  moderately high blood pressure and, 43
  modern medicine and, 39
  mortality rates, medieval Europe, 37–38
  Seventh Day Adventists study, 137
  Super Immunity and increased, 3, 18
  vegetables and, 18, 19, 136
lung cancer, 42, 64, 146
lupus, 70, 168
  nutritional intervention, 169–73
lutein, 16, 33, 146
lycopene, 16, 33, 34, 116, 146
lymphoma, 165

macronutrients, 21, 22, 23–24, 25, 110–29.
  See also carbohydrates; fats, dietary;
    proteins
mango
  in "Clean Fifteen," 166

Mumbai Stuffer, 237
Rainbow Chopped Salad, 206
Tropical Fruit Salad, 209
medical care, 5–8, 39–56
  flu shots, pro and con, 47–52
  influence of commercial interests, 50, 84
  Kaiser Health Foundation study, 5
  lifestyle interventions, 39, 40
  pharmaceuticals and, 39, 40–45, 84
medical foods, 23
medications, 39–45
  all drugs as toxic, 7, 56
  antibiotics, 7, 87–92, 152–53
  antiviral drugs, 52–53
  blood pressure-lowering, 41–43
  for diabetes, 40–41
  flu shots, pro and con, 47–52
  lack of effectiveness, 5–6
  OTC, for colds and flu, 92–96
  risk-to-benefit ratio, 7, 42, 45, 52
Mediterranean diet, 119–20
menu plans, 178–84
micronutrients, 14, 22, 24
  in carbohydrates, 113
  deficiencies of, 21–22
  -dense diet, 59–60
  as determinant of health, 25
  diets low in, viral illness and, 33
  fat necessary for absorption, 25
  fortification of foods and, 22–23
  health benefits, 66
  nutrient density, 27, 69, 131
  revolution, 82–84
millet
  GI and GL of, 112
  resistant starch + fiber in, 114
mushrooms, 13, 23, 69–75, 82
  All-American Spinach with, 220
  anticancer and immune system-
    enhancing, 59, 69–75
  Anticancer Soup, 216
  Better Burgers, 222
  "Cheesy" Kale Soup, 214
  cooking, 71, 74
  Creamy Butternut Squash Soup with,
    215
  Creamy Cruciferous Curry, 225
  Cremini Ratatouille, 226
  dendritic cells and, 72
  Easy Vegetable Pizza, 226
  Green Leafy Moroccan Medley, 228
  Mighty, Stroganoff, 230–31

mushrooms *(continued)*
 nutrient density, 27, 131
 Portobello, and Beans, 231
 Shiitake Watercress Soup, 218
 Super Food Stuffed Peppers, 233
 Sweet Beet Potato Cakes with Strawberry
  sauce, 194
 synergy with greens/onions, 71, 72, 74
 Thai Longevity Stew, 236
 zinc in, 103
mustard greens, 69, 82
 Green Leafy Moroccan Medley, 228
 nutrient density, 131
myrosinase, 67–68

Nakajima, Hiroshi, 30
non-Hodgkin's lymphoma, 57–58, 87
Nrf2, 66
nutritarian diet, 14, 18, 52. *See also* Super
  Foods
 carbs, recommended, 113–14
 carbs, unacceptable, 114–15
 colorful vegetables and, 111
 core concepts review, 129–33
 emphasis on fruits and vegetables, 26,
  28
 fat percentage not important to, 111
 five rules, 130
 foods to avoid, 130
 health equation, 109
 as intervention for viral diseases, 34–35
 men and, 131–32
 overview, 175–78
 questions to ask yourself, 115
 safe percentage of animal products,
  processed foods, 130
 special needs and, 140–42
 vegan vs. near-vegan, 136–39
 women and, 131
nuts, 36, 80
 Apple Berrynut Bites, 238
 as best-high fat food, 116, 118
 calories per ounce, 118
 chocolate nut icing, 244
 Dr. Fuhrman's Food Pyramid and, 28
 health benefits of raw, 117, 118
 nutrient density of, 27, 131
 phytochemical absorption and, 117, 120
 phytochemicals in, 118
 Powerhouse Micro Salad, 206
 recommended daily amount, 120, 177
 roasting, 120–21

servings per day, 130
 Seventh Day Adventists study and, 137
 weight loss and, 120

oats/oatmeal, 113
 Better Burgers, 222
 Chia Cookies, 240
 GI and GL of rolled, 112
 Go Berry Breakfast Bars, 191
 nutrient density, 27
 piecrust, 242–43
 Quick Banana Berry Breakfast to Go, 192
 resistant starch + fiber in rolled, 114
obesity. *See also* weight loss
 foods that promote angiogenesis, 75
 malnutrition and, 35
 nutritional protection from, 52
 pathogenic bacteria, yeasts, and, 91
olive oil, 119–20
 amount recommended daily, 132
 nutrient density, 27
omega-3 fatty acids, 75, 81, 116, 139, 141,
  161–64
omega-6 fatty acids, 116, 161
onions, 13, 82
 All-American Spinach with Mushrooms,
  220
 as angiogenesis inhibitor, 74, 75
 anticancer and immune system-
  enhancing of, 59, 72, 76–77
 Anticancer Soup, 216
 Braised Kale and Squash with Pumpkin
  Seeds, 224
 in "Clean Fifteen," 166
 Goji Chili Stew, 227
 Golden, Morsels, 211
 Green Leafy Moroccan Medley, 228
 nutrient density, 27, 131
 Veggie Scramble, 195
oral cancers, 79
orange(s)
 Cashame Dressing, 200
 Marinated Kale Salad, 204
 nutrient density, 27, 131
 Peanut Ginger Dressing, 200
 Phyto-Blast Breakfast Bowl, 191
 Tropical Fruit Salad, 209
organic foods, 165–67
organosulfides, 19
osteoporosis, 22, 147, 155
ovarian cancer, 60–61, 160
Overdosed America (Abramson), 40

pancreatic cancer, 26, 65, 125
pasta
    amount recommended, 132
    GI and GL of, 112
    Mighty Mushroom Stroganoff, 230–31
    nutrient density, 27
peaches
    pesticides and, 166
    Very Berry Smoothie, 198
peanut butter
    nutrient density, 27
    Peanut Ginger Dressing, 200
    Thai Longevity Stew, 236
peas, 19
    Anticancer Soup, 216
    "Cheesy" Kale Soup, 214
    in "Clean Fifteen," 166
    Creamy Cruciferous Curry, 225
    Mighty Mushroom Stroganoff, 230–31
    nutrient density, 27
    protein content, 122
    as recommended carb, 113
pecans
    Apple Berrynut Bites, 238
    Powerhouse Micro Salad, 206
    Spinach Salad with Strawberry Sesame
        Vinaigrette, 207
pectins, 16, 19
pelagonium, 100
peppers (red or green bell), 19, 75
    Bean Enchiladas, 221
    Cremini Ratatouille, 226
    nutrient density, 27, 131
    pesticides and, 166
    Super Food Stuffed, 233
    Veggie Scramble, 195
pesticides, 164–67
    Dirty Dozen and Clean Fifteen, 166
pharyngitis, 92
phenolic acids, 16, 19
phenylethyl-isothiocyanate (PEITC), 64
phytochemicals, 9, 11–12, 14, 19, 20
    absorption of, 117, 120
    as anti-inflammatory, 127
    as antioxidants, 16
    in coffee, 157
    in mushrooms, 69–70
    synergy and, 72
phytoesterols, 19
phytoestrogens, 159
pineapple
    in "Clean Fifteen," 166

Got Greens Smoothie, 197
Healthy Chocolate Cake, 244
Tropical Fruit Salad, 209
pine nuts, 141
    Pesto Dressing, 201
pistachio nuts, nutrient density, 27, 131
Platt, Cheryl, 169–70
plums, nutrient density, 27, 131
pneumonia, 3, 11
polyphenols, 16, 78
pomegranates/juice, 13, 77–79, 82, 106
    as angiogenesis inhibitor, 75, 77, 78
    anticancer and immune system-
        enhancing of, 59
    benefits, list of, 78–79
    how to open, 78
    nutrient density, 27, 131
    Pomegranate Museli, 192
    Purple Power Smoothie, 198
    Waldorf Blended Salad, 198
Popcorn, Seasoned Kale Chips and, 213
potato (white)
    amount recommended daily, 132
    GI and GL of, 112
    nutrient density, 27
    pesticides and, 166
    resistant starch + fiber in, 114
pregnancy
    folate during, 150–51
    folic acid supplements, 148, 149, 150
    processed meats and child cancer, 150
proanthocyanins, 16
probiotics, 89, 106, 151–54
    supplements, indications for, 153, 172
    who should avoid supplements,
        153–54
processed foods, 4, 14–16, 15
    avoiding, 109
    breakfast cereal, 109, 113
    deficiencies of, 16, 17, 20
    disease and, 38
    Dr. Fuhrman's Food Pyramid and, 28
    foods to eliminate, 177
    fortification of, 22
    high GI effect of, 113
    in modern diet, 14–16, 22, 23, 35, 109
    oils as, 118
    questions to ask yourself, 115
    safe percentage of daily, 130, 131–32
    salt intake and, 156
    soy and, 160–61
    waste products and, 109–10

prostate cancer
  folic acid and increased risk, 149
  IGF-1 and, 126, 127
  nutritional anticancer agents, 64, 78,
    160, 161
  pesticides and, 165
  servings of vegetables per week to
    reduce risk, 64
proteins, 121–29
  aging and, 123
  American over-consumption, 121, 129
  amino acids and, 127
  amount recommended daily, 140
  animal vs. plant-based, 121–24
  best plant protein, 118, 127–29
  content of common plant foods, 122
  digestive impairment and, 142
  excess, problems of, 123
  high-protein, low carb diet, 138
  IGF-1 and, 124–27
  inhibitors, 19
  maximum muscle mass weekly and, 123
  sources for higher requirements, 141
  soy, 128, 159–61
  supplements of, 123
psoriasis, 168
pumpkin seeds, 81
  Braised Kale and Squash with, 224
  zinc in, 103

quercetin, 16, 172
quince, 75
quinoa
  as recommended carb, 113
  Super Food Stuffed Peppers, 233

radishes, 69
raspberries, 79–80
  Detox Green Tea, 197
  nutrient density, 27, 131
  Very Berry Smoothie, 198
Ratatouille, Cremini, 226
resveratrol, 75, 101–2
rheumatoid arthritis, 70, 168
  nutritional intervention for, 168, 169
riboflavin, 33, 34
Ricci, Diana, 37
rice, black, 75
  anthocyanins in, 105
  Forbidden Rice Pudding, 190
rice, brown
  GI and GL of, 112

protein content, 122
  resistant starch + fiber in, 114
rice, white
  GI and GL of rolled, 112
  resistant starch + fiber, 114
rice, wild
  as recommended carb, 113
  zinc in, 103
ROS (reactive oxygen species), 66
rutin, 16

salad dressings, 177
  from nuts and seeds, 116–17, 120
  recipes, 199–201, 203, 205, 207
salads
  blended, 57, 68, 170, 172, 198
  one large per day, 129, 130, 175
  recipes, 202–9
salsa, Black Bean and Corn, 210
salt (sodium), 154–56
  alternatives, 156
  avoiding, 172
  reducing, fatigue and, 141
SARS (severe acute respiratory syndrome), 4
sea salt, 156
seeds, 36, 80–82
  ALA in, 162
  anticancer and immune system-
    enhancing of, 59, 161
  as best-high fat food, 116, 118
  calories per ounce, 118
  Dr. Fuhrman's Food Pyramid and, 28
  health benefits of raw, 117, 118
  nutrient density, 27, 131
  percentage of modern diet, 15, 23
  phytochemical absorption and, 117, 120
  phytochemicals in, 118
  recommended daily amount, 130, 177
  roasting, 120–21
  Seventh Day Adventists study and, 137
  as super food, 82
  Super Seed Oatmeal, 193
selenium, 17, 33, 34
  foods high in, 81
sesame seeds, 81, 82, 119
  Eggplant Hummus, 211
  nutrient density, 27, 131
  Orange Cashame Dressing, 200
  Strawberry Sesame Vinaigrette, 207
  toasting, 208
  Triple Treat Cabbage Salad dressing, 208
  zinc in, 103

Seventh Day Adventists study, 137
sinusitis, 5, 6, 11
smoothie recipes, 196–98
snow peas: Thai Longevity Stew, 236
soft drinks, 15, 130
    nutrient density, 27
soup recipes, 214–19
soybeans, 133
    as angiogenesis inhibitor, 75
    phytochemicals in, 159
    protein in, 141
soy protein, 128, 159–61
    amino acids and, 128
    breast cancer and, 159–60
    IGF-1 and, 128
    processed, avoiding, 160–61
Spaghetti Squash Primavera, 232
spinach
    All-American. with Mushrooms, 220
    as angiogenesis inhibitor, 75
    Apple Berrynut Bites, 238
    folate in, 148
    Got Greens Smoothie, 197
    nutrient density, 27, 131
    pesticides and, 166
    protein content, 122
    Purple Power Smoothie, 198
    Salad with Strawberry Sesame
        Vinaigrette, 207
    Veggie Scramble, 195
squash, winter, 19
    Acorn Squash Supreme, 220
    Braised Kale and, with Pumpkin Seeds,
        224
    Creamy Butternut, Soup with
        Mushrooms, 215
    as recommended carb, 113
Standard American Diet, 15
    angiogenesis (and tumor growth) and,
        75
    disease risk of Americans and, 30
    food pyramid, 28
    gross deficiencies of, 16, 23, 31, 35
    processed foods in, 14–16, 109
    reduction of immunity and, 4, 6
    sodium levels in, 154
    sweeteners in, 15
stanols, 119
sterols (plant), 118, 119
stew recipes, 227, 229, 236
stomach cancer, 26
    dietary anticancer agents, 66, 71

pesticides and, 165
salt intake and, 155
strawberry(ies), 80
    Apple Berrynut Bites, 238
    Detox Green Tea, 197
    nutrient density, 27, 131
    pesticides and, 166
    Purple Power Smoothie, 198
    sauce, 194
    Spinach Salad with, Sesame Vinaigrette,
        207
Streptococcus pneumoniae, 65
stroke, 14, 38, 46
    beta-blockers and increased risk, 42
    hypertension and, 154
    nutritional protection from, 36, 83
    salt intake and, 154–55
sulforaphane, 63, 64
summer squash, 113
sunflower seeds, 81, 82
    nutrient density, 27, 131
    protein in, 122, 141
    zinc in, 103
Super Foods, 13, 21, 80
    Top Super Foods, 82
    Top 30 Super Foods, 26, 131
Super Food Stuffed Peppers, 233
Super Immunity, 1, 3, 8–9, 12–13, 14, 18,
        19, 36, 59. See also immune system;
        nutritarian diet
    aggregation of super foods and, 82
    autoimmune diseases and, 167–73
    five rules, 130
    GOMBBS, 83
    menu plans, 178–84
    nutrient density scores, 27, 131
    proteins and, 129
    scientific credentials, 21–23
    super foods, 13, 21, 80
    Top Super Foods, 82
    Top 30 Super Foods, 26, 131
    vitamin D and, 104
    whole foods vs. extracts, 13–14
supplements, 58, 144–51
    autoimmune diseases protocol, 172
    beta-carotene caution, 146–47
    copper caution, 151
    DHA and EPA, 138, 172
    fish oil, 161, 163–64
    folic acid caution, 145
    healthy diet preferred to, 151
    iodine, 139, 144

supplements *(continued)*
  multivitamin/multimineral supplement,
    troublesome elements of, 144–54
  probiotics, 153–54
  taurine, 142
  vitamin A caution, 145, 147
  vitamin B12, 138, 139
  vitamin D, 139
  vitamin E caution, 145
  zinc, 139, 144
sweeteners
  angiogenesis (and tumor growth) and,
    75
  avoiding, 130, 140, 172
  in modern diet, 15, 35
sweet potato
  in "Clean Fifteen," 166
  GI and GL of, 112
  as recommended carb, 113
  resistant starch + fiber in, 114
  Sweet Beet Potato Cakes with Strawberry
    sauce, 194
  Swiss Chard and, Gratin, 234
Swiss chard, 19
  and Sweet Potato Gratin, 234

tannins, 78
taurine, 142
tempeh, 128
  Swiss Chard and Sweet Potato
    Gratin, 234
terpenes (isoprenoids), 19
Thai Longevity Stew, 236
tofu, 128
  Brussels sprouts Polonaise, 224
  nutrient density of, 27
  Russian Vinaigrette Dressing, 201
  Veggie Scramble, 195
tomatoes, 82
  as angiogenesis inhibitor, 75
  Bisque, 219
  Black Bean and Corn Salsa, 210
  Cremini Ratatouille, 226
  Goji Chili Stew, 227
  Green Leafy Moroccan Medley, 228
  Home-Style Ketchup, 212
  Italian Stuffer, 237
  nutrient density, 27, 131
  as recommended carb, 113
  Spaghetti Squash Primavera, 232
  Super Food Stuffed Peppers, 233
  Veggie Scramble, 195

toxins
  in animal products, 165
  pesticides, 164–67
  phytochemicals and resistance to, 20
  transcription factor, 66–67
triglycerides
  foods to avoid, 109
  raw seeds and nuts for, 117
trigonelline, 157
turmeric, 75, 172
turnip greens, 69
  nutrient density, 131
turnips, 62
tyrosol esters, 19

ulcerative colitis, 168
UTIs (urinary tract infections), 6, 87–88

vegan diet, 177
  autoimmune diseases and, 168, 172
  B12 deficiency and, 138, 139
  EPA and DHA deficiency and, 138–39
  IGF-1 and lowered levels, 128
  iodine and zinc deficiencies, 139, 144
  Seventh Day Adventists study, 137
  vegan diet vs. near-vegan, 136–39
vegetable(s), 15, 16, 17–18
  amount recommended daily, 177
  blood test for alpha-carotene and,
    17–18
  cancer and, 19, 61–62
  colors and, 17, 18, 33, 111
  Creamy Cruciferous Curry, 225
  cruciferous, 36, 62–69, 75
  Dr. Fuhrman's Food Pyramid and, 28
  Easy, Pizza, 226
  green, 13, 25–26, 33, 61–62, 71
  immune system and, 26, 59
  longevity and, 18, 19, 136
  micronutrients in, 25, 27
  in modern diet, 15, 23
nutrient density scores, 27, 131
  organic and pesticides, 164–67
  raw, 36, 68
  Spaghetti Squash Primavera, 232
viruses, 8
  bronchitis and, 86
  colds and flu, 85–107
  cruciferous vegetables as antivirals, 65–67
  elderberry extract treatment, 104–5
  etiology of, 30–31
  herbal treatment, 99–100

maintaining CNA and, 31
micronutrients and severity of, 33, 34
mucus color and, 86
mutation dangers, 32–36
neuropathy following illness, 34
nutritarian diet as intervention, 34–35
reducing exposure to, 31, 54–55
sinusitis and sinus congestion, 86
sore throats and, 86
vulnerability to, nutrition and,
    29–32, 34
vitamin A, 22
    supplement caution, 145, 147
vitamin B12, 138, 139
vitamin C, 13, 17, 22, 36
    as antioxidant, 67
    for colds and flu, 98–99
vitamin D, 22, 36, 52, 139
    for autoimmune diseases, 172
    for colds and flu, 104
vitamin E, 13, 17, 34
    as antioxidant, 67
    facts about, 81–82
    foods high in, 81
    supplement caution, 145
vitamin K, 89
vitamins and minerals, 14, 16, 20. See also
    specific types

Waldorf Blended Salad, 198
walnuts, 119, 141
    ALA in, 161
    Better Burgers, 222
    Black Cherry Sorbet, 239
    Chunky Blueberry, Sorbet, 241
    Cinnamon Apple Omega Milk, 196
    ETs in, 118
    Healthy Chocolate Cake, 244
    nutrient density, 27, 131
    Waldorf Blended Salad, 198
    Wild Blueberry Hot Breakfast, 195
warts, 65
watercress, 69, 82
    nutrient density, 27, 131
    Nutri-Green Salad with Black Fig
        Dressing, 205
    Shiitake, Soup, 218
watermelon, in "Clean Fifteen," 166

weight loss, 1, 2
    anti-angiogenic foods and nutrients
        for, 75
    foods to avoid, 109
    greens and, 129
    ineffective methods, 6
    raw seeds and nuts for, 117, 120
    super immunity foods and, 6
weight maintenance, 141–42
Westfall, Ondria, 175
West Nile virus, 3
wheat, avoiding, 172
wheat berries, as recommended carb, 113
white foods/white bread, 109
    amount recommended daily, 132
    avoiding, 130
    GI and GL of, 112
    nutrient density, 27
    resistant starch + fiber in, 114
    rule and rhyme for, 115
    waste products and, 109–10
whole grains
    Dr. Fuhrman's Food Pyramid and, 28
    GI and GL of wheat, 112
    Healthy Chocolate Cake, 244
    nutrient density, 27
    protein content of bread, 122
    as recommended carb, 113
    resistant starch + fiber in wheat, 114

yeasts, 91

Zabransky, Irene, 57–58
zeaxanthin, 16
zinc, 33, 102
    for colds and flu, 102–4
    foods high in, 81, 103
    supplements, 139, 144
    vegan diet and, 139
zucchini
    Anticancer Soup, 216
    Creamy Butternut Squash Soup with
        Mushrooms, 215
    Cremini Ratatouille, 226
    Goji Chili Stew, 227
    Spaghetti Squash Primavera, 232
    Super Food Stuffed Peppers, 233
    Tangy White Beans and, 235

Scan this code with your smartphone

to be instantly linked to *Super Immunity* bonus materials and other healthy living books and information.

You can also text keyword **IMMUNITY** to **READIT** (732348) to be sent a link to Elixir, a mobile website.

elixir: your source for healthy living

brought to you by HarperOne

Made in the USA
Middletown, DE
20 September 2022

10875969R00169